Midwives' Emotional Care of Women becoming Mothers

Midwives' Emotional Care of Women becoming Mothers

By

Sue Barker

CAMBRIDGE
SCHOLARS
PUBLISHING

Midwives' Emotional Care of Women becoming Mothers,
by Sue Barker

This book first published 2011

Cambridge Scholars Publishing

12 Back Chapman Street, Newcastle upon Tyne, NE6 2XX, UK

British Library Cataloguing in Publication Data
A catalogue record for this book is available from the British Library

ISBN (10): 1-4438-2730-4, ISBN (13): 978-1-4438-2730-0

TABLE OF CONTENTS

Acknowledgements vii

Introduction 1

Chapter One 5
What is Motherhood?

Chapter Two 21
Who Supports Women becoming Mothers?

Chapter Three 45
What is Emotional Care?

Chapter Four 69
Midwives' Emotional Care of Women becoming Mothers

Chapter Five 97
What are the Experiences of Midwives giving Emotional Support?

Chapter Six 127
What is Emotion Work?

Chapter Seven 141
How Might Emotional Support Help Women on their Journey
to Motherhood?

References 161

ACKNOWLEDGEMENTS

I primarily thank all the midwives who took part in this study, without you there would be no study – thank you for sharing your experiences; it was an honour and privilege to hear about your emotional work.

Thank you to my supervisors for your patience, encouragement and commitment to me and the study. Professor Jo Alexander, your guidance, particularly in those early tentative days before a research proposal had been developed and your faith in my ability to undertake a study like this, although I did not always believe you, increased my motivation and my self esteem. Professor Les Todres, your calm, trusting, patient benevolence allowed me to follow Jo's advice and to 'smell the flowers'! Associate Professor Fran Biley who joined Les in my supervision in those long dark days of writing up the study, your challenging and guidance were just what I needed when I needed it. Thank you all.

There are many who have encouraged and supported me with undertaking this study including my midwifery and adult nursing colleagues and I will continue to be grateful and appreciative of them. There are, though, some who need to be mentioned for their particular assistance with writing this book. I am particularly grateful to Professor Jonathan Parker for his critical reading of my writing and to Greta Richardson for her assistance with my idiosyncratic grammar.

Along with all those mentioned above I must also acknowledge my ever tolerant husband, Julian, who has suffered take away meals and has had to endure social interactions with his computer games instead of my scintillating conversation!

Thank you.

INTRODUCTION

This book owes its genesis to a number of factors and offers the journey of understanding of its author. I have spent many years working as a mental health nurse, at times, working with women who were suffering significant levels of mental ill-health during pregnancy and the early days, months and years after the birth of their baby. I have also worked with women who were 'incarcerated' in the old mental hospitals due to 'odd' behaviour after having their babies. This was many years ago, but, by the time I was nursing them, they were unable to return to what might be considered a normal life. The focus on community care starting in the 1970s and the new treatments available were, in many ways, too late for them as indicated by Enoch Powell's White Paper in 1962 (NHS 1962).

I have also worked with people who have been diagnosed with the psychiatric label of severe personality disorder. When we were able to find out about their early life experiences, we found many had poor maternal attachments which they were not able to resolve and, therefore, adopted what we perceived as maladaptive coping strategies.

My concern for those who experience emotional distress, mental distress or mental illness at such a vulnerable time for them and their baby was increased further when I, too, developed depression during both of my pregnancies and into the first year of my children's lives. I was fortunate in the care I received from the mental health services and both I and my children have thrived. Both my children are high- achieving adults of whom I am immensely proud. This is not, though, the situation for all who develop emotional or psychological problems at this time.

When I was offered the opportunity to undertake a PhD, exploring how I could help women at this significant stage was my first desire. As with any research proposal, I undertook a literature review and found many studies on the treatment of postnatal depression, its aetiology and the risk factors. I therefore had some understanding of what happens when women are diagnosed and treated by GPs, psychologists or psychiatric services. The literature also led to some concerns, as it suggested that not all women experiencing emotional distress were identified and treated, either by primary care or mental health services. It seemed pertinent, therefore, to find out what happened to these women who were not 'picked up'. Likewise, this book has the same focus.

The only sensible way to explore the emotional care or support these women were given was to conduct a literature search on the emotional care given to women who experience 'normal' transitions. Armed with this knowledge, I could then look at how this could be improved, so that all women who experienced emotional distress at this time could be helped. This was the point where my literature search met a dead-end. I eventually found a paper by Hunter (2001), which informed me that my lack of success in finding studies in this area was due to the lack of studies, not my lack of ability.

Whilst this was a relief on the one hand, it became a pivotal moment in my PhD work. After discussion with my supervisors it was clear that, to progress, I needed to explore whether women were supported emotionally at this time and, if so, who supported them and what this support looked like. Through discussion with colleagues, meetings with maternity service providers and considering the literature, it became apparent that the health professional who had the most contact with women on this journey was the midwife. The educational literature, their professional bodies and governmental policies all appeared to indicate that midwives provided support for women through pregnancy and into the early days after the birth of the baby.

It became apparent that there was a need to establish if midwives actually were providing emotional support to women through their transition to motherhood and, if so, what it looked like. Given that there was limited information available on this type of care in midwifery, a qualitative approach to exploring the area appeared appropriate. Given my worldview, psychological education and the lack of clarity of the concepts involved, I needed to use an exploratory, yet scientific, method.

There were a number of qualitative approaches that initially appeared worth exploring. Ethnography, grounded theory, narrative and phenomenological approaches, all to a greater or lesser degree, could be considered scientific and all offered a method for exploring uncharted areas for discovery. After much reading, and with supervision, I finally settled on a descriptive phenomenological approach. There were a number of reasons for this, but probably the strongest was my psychological background - it made sense to me!

Amedeo Giorgi (1979), a psychologist by background too, with an extensive understanding of Husserl's phenomenological philosophy, had grappled with the need to stay loyal to his background, as well as to Husserl. This led to his development of a research approach called psychological phenomenology. It is descriptive phenomenology, but adapted to facilitate the psychological researcher.

Husserl's philosophical phenomenology had developed to allow the philosopher to explore their own lifeworld through transcendental phenomenological reduction. He did accept, though, that phenomenological reduction could occur at lower levels than a transcendental state, but this was the aim. What Giorgi's approach facilitated was the ability of researchers to gain an understanding of other people's lifeworlds by analysing their detailed descriptions of experiences in a phenomenologically reduced state. Giorgi did not make the same claims for the findings as Husserl. Husserl was trying to see the 'thing itself' (noema) without perceptual interference (noesis); the universal essential features (Husserl 1970b). Giorgi's claim was that phenomenological researchers could establish generally applicable features through psychological phenomenology (Giorgi and Giorgi 2003).

Using this approach I set out to establish if midwives normally gave emotional support to women on their journey to motherhood and, if they did, what it looked like. I collected data through individual interviews; these were unstructured. I asked midwives to describe their experience of offering emotional support to women. The midwives seemed very happy to describe their experiences of emotionally supporting women and shared some quite emotive interactions. Quotes from these interviews are mainly in chapters four and five.

My literature review initially was quite small, as I was searching for specific literature on midwives' emotional support, but after completing the analysis of the interview data I found a number of areas where there was literature pertinent to my study. There was a great deal of literature on information-giving and breast-feeding. Also, as I have continued to work on literature in this area, Hunter and colleagues have dramatically increased the research in emotional labour / work of midwives.

This book is based on the literature reviews and findings of my study, initially conceived as 'how do midwives give emotional support to women on their journey to motherhood?. I hope I have been able to add to the knowledge base of what emotional support is, how it appears to be part of emotional care and the complexities of how it is provided.

CHAPTER ONE

WHAT IS MOTHERHOOD?

Introduction

This chapter explores what motherhood is and how women experience it. The underpinning political ideologies along with generally accepted myths of motherhood are discussed. Women's experiences of becoming mothers are explored later in the chapter, which concludes with a consideration of women's goal to be a 'good mother'.

> Mother n. 1. Female parent 7. Hence ~ hood n.
> Motherly a. having or showing the good (esp. tender or kind) qualities of a mother (Sykes 1982:660),

> "Becoming a mother affects your life in ways you cannot even begin to imagine. It is one of the most dramatic and profound personal transformations a woman can ever experience. It will change your way of thinking in areas you believed had nothing to do with mothering. It will change how you view the world. It will change how you relate to other people. It will change how you see your past, present and future.
>
> Your experiences will take you on a breathtaking journey as intense in joy and euphoria as in pain and confusion"
> (Leonhardt-Lupa 1995:1).

What is motherhood?

Motherhood has been described as the ultimate achievement and fulfilment of a woman's life, but others see it as an ultimate example of female oppression (Marchant 2004).

Motherhood has been said to be impossible to define in any helpful way (Ball 1994) but Marchant (2004:74) offers the definition "motherhood implies the act of having given birth". This simple definition corresponds highly with the dictionary definition, but it is important, when developing a detailed understanding, to consider what it means to the person experiencing it (Ball 1994). Motherhood, when considering more closely the experiences of women, may be a process involving both physical and psychological changes through pregnancy, giving birth and nurturing a child, rather than just the end point of birth. It is also acknowledged that birthing can be described as a process, rather than an event. It is recognised that motherhood involves strong emotions alongside physical, sexual and spiritual changes (Ball 1994, Page and McCandlish 2006, Atkinson 2006). Whilst the major physical changes may not occur for women who become mothers without pregnancy and giving birth, there are still many social and psychological changes that take place for them.

The term motherhood can be seen as problematic, if accepted as 'the act of having given birth' as, within our society, there are many women who undertake the role of 'being a mother' without having given birth. Hence the focus in the literature has been on mothering, instead of motherhood (Marchant 2004). Mothering can be seen as a way of caring, exhibited through altruistic, undemanding, selfless love (Marchant 2004). Motherhood can therefore be seen as the state, status or role of being or becoming a mother and mothering as the actions in response to it, such as loving and caring. "Mothering is an intimate kind of caring" (Rothman 2000: 9).

Through our society's political ideologies, motherhood can be seen to be promoted as an idealised state where mothers appear unrealistically happy and healthy, and the expectation of emotional fulfilment in motherhood has led to some disillusionment (Magill-Coerden 2006). It could also be suggested that the origins of this disillusionment, unhappiness or something that could be labelled depression, are in the nature of care provision – its medicalisation (Littlewood and McHugh 1997).

In the past, motherhood has defined women and their activities - it was their status, it was who they were. Feminists fought against this to gain choices and opportunities for women, but this has led to an even more unacceptable definition of motherhood (Rothman 2000). Instead of motherhood being a status, it has become an activity, a service or work. Rothman suggests this is reducing the enormity of the experience which, in turn, could have an impact on the whole of society. If motherhood can be seen as work or a job, it could be suggested that the loving care that supports it can also be a commodity that is bought and sold. Certainly Hochschild (2003) recognises this as already occurring in her book, *The Commercialisation of Intimate Life*.

Political ideologies influencing motherhood

Motherhood has been part of political ideology since the mid-twentieth century (Magill-Coerden 2006). A political ideology is the power-base for the society, influencing its attitudes, values and morality. This is sometimes referred to as hegemony, which means ruling or leadership by one state over the available others. Hegemony does not necessarily refer to coercive control, despite frequently being seen as such; it can have an underpinning or implicit impact on states or societies. Political ideologies in western societies can be seen more, though, as cultural hegemonies, as established by the Marxist movement. Marxists suggest cultural hegemony occurs where there are differing classes or groups within a society and the 'ruling' class or group establishes the cultural 'norms' for that society (MIA 2010). The less powerful groups then implicitly accept the values and morality of the 'ruling' group without explicit consideration. Political ideologies can therefore be seen as underpinning the attitudes, values and morality of a society and are accepted, without thinking, as the 'right way to be'.

Rothman (2000) suggests there are three political ideologies that apply to motherhood in the US - patriarchy, technology and capitalism. These three political ideologies can be seen in most Western cultures but perhaps are more distinct in the US, as the socialist approaches of some of the European countries are unacceptable there. Rothman (2000) identifies an ideology as a worldview which influences not only how people interact with each other, but also how a person views their own body.

The ideology of patriarchy can lead women to believe they are lesser human beings than men, their views and abilities are less important and less valuable. In her discussion of patriarchy in the US, Rothman is not referring to male dominance; she believes it is the patriarchal kinship that is the foundation of this (patriarchal) ideology. The male, or father, relationship is core in the society and expresses this as "children are born to men out of women" (Rothman 2000: 15). This can be seen in the way in which people express their kinship and their explanations of reproduction. It still appears acceptable to refer to procreation in the US and UK as men's seed growing in women's bodies. Men, in the patriarchal ideology, can be seen to control procreation; the seed of life comes from them. Women in this culture are expected to be virgins at marriage and are controlled through pregnancy, to ensure the protection of the man's seed. Evidence of a patriarchal society can be seen in the naming of children in the US and UK: children usually receive their family name from the man.

The technology ideology, which has grown out of the Industrial Revolution, changed not only the tools available, but also the way people think about themselves and the world (Rothman 2000), although others, such as Whitbeck, prefer to label this the economy ideology. Within this ideology there is a focus on 'making' rather than 'doing', it is the goal or output that is valued with the "rational pursuit of efficiency" (Rothman 2000: 30). The woman's body and the baby become a resource that can be substituted, or bought and sold. This pursuit of efficiency can be seen in the medicalisation of becoming a mother.

"The ideology of technology dehumanises people by encouraging a mechanical self image – people viewing themselves as machines. Capitalism adds that, not only is the baby a collection of parts, its parts become commodities. In the United States the essential fluids of life – blood, milk, and semen- are all for sale" (Rothman 2000: 39). The paternal ideology, which has been a core ideology in the majority of civilisations for most centuries, guides women to see themselves and their functions, abilities and experiences as being less valuable than men's. With the huge societal changes in western cultures, starting with the Industrial Revolution, this technology ideology emerged which appears to subjugate, not only women, but all human experience. Alongside the technology ideology has been the development of capitalism. Capitalism can be seen to be influential in all western societies as not only a political and economic approach, but also a distinct belief system: an ideology.

Rothman (2000; 39) suggests the capitalism ideology leads to the "commodification of children and the proletarianisation of motherhood". This commodification of 'properties' associated with motherhood, can be seen to lead to people to declaring, and at times demanding, property 'rights'. Although it is politically unacceptable to state children are properties that can be owned in the US or UK, there are 'rights' attributed to them which can be seen to be similar to property rights or legislation. Men and women believe they have the right to have a baby or the right to terminate a pregnancy. There is still legal debate and there have been a number of court cases where the right of the woman to terminate a pregnancy and the prospective father's right to the foetus have been conducted.

There appears to be a strong link between the technology and capitalism ideologies in relationship to motherhood. Both can be seen to lead to a more medicalised experience of the transition to motherhood. With technological advances there are many interventions now that can substitute parts of procreation, such as fallopian tubes and breasts and others to alter the transitional experience, such as amniocentesis and caesarean sections. The capitalist underlying ideological approach to rights, including the right to 'sue' associated with motherhood and fatherhood, promote the acquisition of the elements of technology they choose, in order to control their bodies and their babies.

This very brief exploration of the prevalent ideologies in western societies has mostly focused on how these belief systems affect the individual, but there are also other societal influences in motherhood. Within the UK, most health and social care is provided by the State, which means the pervasive ideology in the UK is not necessarily the capitalist one in terms of health and social care. There is, though, evidence to support all three of the ideologies discussed here, especially when considering the medicalisation of midwifery care.

Medical-political ideology of childbirth

There has been a lot of discussion surrounding the area of the medicalisation of child- birth within midwifery services, research and in academia. There has certainly been a dramatic increase in the medicalisation of the journey to motherhood over the last century which may have prompted these discussions. The twentieth century saw 15% of births occurring in institutions in 1927, increasing to 24% by 1932 and 45% by 1944 (Leap and Hunter 1993). This had increased to 64% by 1952 (Rhodes 1995). The National Health Service was introduced in 1948 and midwifery services were included in this. By the 1960's there was a call for all births to be in hospital and in the 1970's and '80's, with increasing medical interventions available and a consumer- led health care, this gained momentum (Peel report 1970, Court report 1976, Welburn 1980 cited in Littlewood and McHugh 1997). This has developed with professional midwives and obstetricians taking women through the process and increasingly using technological screening of both mother and baby. This can be seen to be leading women to feel that they are objects being processed through a factory (Rhodes 1995) and it has led to an increase in psychological problems for women (Littlewood and McHugh 1997).

There appear to be two major political discourses in motherhood in the UK, through which the disjunction between expectations and experiences can be explored; they are the discourses of medicine and nature. The medical discourse can be seen in the professionalisation or expert-led maternity care (Littlewood and McHugh 1997), which is underpinned by the technology ideology. The nature discourse establishes becoming a mother as natural or instinctual (Miller 2007), which can be seen in the political ideological stance (Magill-Coerden 2006) taken in the UK, and is closely related to a more paternalistic ideology. Despite this dichotomy, the paternalistic ideology could arguably be said to underpin both discourses as professionalism and medicine have a predominantly masculine approach (Morrison 1992). Miller (2007:337) labels both these views the "unrealistic assumptions embedded in gendered discourses that pattern women's lives".

Given the Marxists' understanding of cultural hegemony and the dominant political ideologies, it can easily be seen how women, whether pregnant, new mothers or midwives would accept the medical-political ideology and submit themselves to professional control. If women accept the medical-political ideology with both the professional and nature discourses it can easily be recognised that women may experience cognitive dissonance and emotional turmoil at this significant time in their lives.

The women's movement in the second half of the twentieth century sought to deal with the inequalities that women experienced, due to the paternal ideology underpinning most western societies. The ideologies of technology, capitalism and paternity do not appear to be mutually exclusive. Despite the feminist impact on legislation and education, their efforts appear to have only intensified the contentions associated with motherhood (DiQuinzio 1999). Feminists have tried to conceptualise motherhood in a way that is emancipatory, but which at the same time addresses the needs and desire of both mother and child. In the US, mothering is a contentious issue, not least for feminists as they struggle with a monolithic view. Some have argued that motherhood is oppressive, and others that it leads to fulfilment and a sense of identify (DiQuinzio 1999).

Despite these debates and discussions, there is general agreement that there are social expectations of mothers – those who experience motherhood (Marchant 2004, Magill-Cuerden 2006, Miller 2007). Magill-Cuerden (2006) states that, to be a 'good parent' the person needs to conform to social expectations. Marchant (2004:75), highlighting this, presents a table of what are considered to be socially normal and deviant behaviours attributed to mothers. To be considered normal, women are expected to be maternal, home-centred, care about their families and men, controlled by their bodies, inferior to men and submissive. Deviant women are those who reject the caring role and are career-orientated, not accepting an inferior position or bodily limits, and are over assertive. Society's concept, outlined by Magill-Cuerden (2006), of a mother is very similar to this, but perhaps more exaggerated. Normal mothers are controlled by their bodies and are emotionally unstable. They are also, paradoxically, expected to be child like at the same time as nest-builders with the urge to care. Socially deviant mothers struggle with childbirth, are unwilling to give up their past life and expect partners to share responsibility. This is very clearly supported by the paternalistic ideology (Rothman 2000).

The stereotypical characteristics listed above are what DiQuinzio (1999) has labelled 'essential motherhood' and states that it puts women in a subjugated position. The paternalistic, technological and capitalist ideologies are enacted in western societies in an individualist manner. This overarching individualist approach identifies each individual as unique; they are objective and can make their own choices based on the resources available to them. Therefore, each individual makes their individual decisions based on their personally determined desires and needs. If all mothers and mothers-to-be are expected to conform to a predetermined stereotype, they cannot be considered individual and are always, therefore, subjective. The expectation to be individualist and conformist is the paradox of the politics of mothering expressed by DiQuinzio (1999). She does, though, offer a way forward, in her suggestion that a politic of mothering could involve a movement between contradictory positions accepting different ways of being, whilst at the same time recognising there are some common needs.

The dissonance associated with cultural hegemony discussed above may be seen to present the experience of motherhood in a rather negative way, with women encouraged to have certain expectations that cannot be achieved and immense societal pressure on them. The reader, though, can be reassured that, although the majority of women experience what is labelled the 'baby blues' in the first week after the birth (Lawrie et al 2002), for many, the experience of becoming a mother is a positive one (Fullerton 1997, Green and Kafetsios 1997).

Myths of motherhood

Barnes and Balber (2007) highlight the myths associated with motherhood and parenthood and guide their readers to more realistic expectations. They write "Babies may embody all the magic, innocence and wonderment of a fairy tale. But the realities of pregnancy, childbirth and the postpartum period can be a very different story" (Barnes and Balber 2007: 8). The myths of parenthood include 'all women "glow" during pregnancy', 'having a baby can save a strained marriage', 'children are destined to repeat their parents' mistakes', 'life will not be that different once the baby arrives', 'the maternal instinct', 'maternal bonding', 'the average baby' and 'the perfect parent'. They state that each of these is a myth, as each may apply in some part to some parents, but these things do not occur in everyone spontaneously.

The myths explored by Barnes and Balber and the advice they go on to offer prospective parents, highlight again the social nature of parenthood. Whereas Magill-Cuerden (2006) and Marchant (2004) acknowledge the social expectations and identify how difficult it is for a mother to be recognised as acceptable if she does not fulfil these, Barnes and Balber (2007) suggest women have choices. They assume that women can grasp the individualist approach and make objective decisions.

Barnes and Balber (2007) appear to suggest women can put on one side the acknowledged stereotypical expectations which are less clearly defined in contemporary society. They are attempting to lead those on the journey to parenthood to develop what they would consider to be more realistic expectations of themselves. They suggest parenting is about trial and error and write of the 'good enough' parent.

From this brief overview, motherhood can be seen to be a process, as well as an event. The event is the giving birth, which is in itself a process, and the processes of physical and psychological changes through pregnancy and birth to the early days of being a mother. All of these are experienced within a political and social environment, which has clear expectations of the woman.

Despite this, understanding is limited unless the women's lived experiences are also considered. To gain a more in-depth understanding of motherhood, becoming and being a mother, there is the need to explore the experiences of women at this time (Ball 1994).

The experiences of women becoming mothers

Most research in this area has been undertaken using a qualitative methodology, but not the same methodology. Studies have used a variety of approaches, including narrative analysis of a longitudinal study (Miller 2007), content analysis (Cronin 2003), phenomenology (Bondas and Eriksson 2001) and grounded theory (Barclay et al 1997). Studies have also been conducted in different countries: UK (Miller 2007), Ireland (Cronin 2003), Finland (Bondas and Eriksson 2001) and Australia (Barclay et al 1997). They can all, though, offer some insight into the phenomenon of how women experience becoming a mother, and those identified above will be explored in chronological order of being undertaken.

A total of fifty-five women in nine focus groups were asked about their experiences of becoming a mother in Australia (Barclay et al 1997). The core category identified was labelled 'becoming a mother'; all the other categories fed into it. There were six other categories: 'working it out', 'alone', 'realising', 'loss', 'unready', and 'drained'. Many adjectives typified each of these categories. For example, for 'alone' the suggestions offered were: isolating, trapped, suffering, confused, vulnerable, being there, feeling supported, safe, frightened, resentful.

The core category of 'becoming a mother', offered the story line for the phenomenon. Despite biologically becoming a mother, the women did not appear to become a mother emotionally and personally until sometime afterwards (Barclay et al 1997). When the women recognised the impact of being a mother, it came as a shock. Eventually, the women tuned in to their babies as they worked out how to be a mother. The social process was identified as both maturational and developmental (Barclay et al 1997).

Forty women's experiences of pregnancy were explored using Colaizzi's phenomenological approach (Bondas and Eriksson 2001). Colaizzi's approach involved a systematic analysis of peoples 'lived' experiences of a given phenomenon; in this case the phenomenon was pregnancy. Pregnancy is a particularly significant time emotionally for women, as they are said to gain higher scores on the Edinburgh Post Natal Depression Scale (EPNDS) in the antenatal period (Evans et al 2001). There are, though, many concerns with using this scale within clinical practice (Adams 2002). A systematic review of depression perinatally offers a prevalence rate of major or minor depression of up to 12.9% (Gavin et al 2005). Despite this being lower than the rate at three months post-natally (19.2% Gavin et al 2005), it is still of significant concern.

Bondas and Eriksson (2001) found ten emerging themes in the women's experiences of pregnancy, which were clustered into three categories. The category of 'the perfect baby' included the themes of promoting the health of the unborn baby, health as no longer taken for granted and changing health behaviours. The category of 'an altered mode of being' included the themes: changing body, variations in mood, ill-health as part of being pregnant and worries. The third category was 'striving for family communion' which incorporated the themes of the evolving significance of the baby, dreams, expectations and planning and changing relationships.

The essence or invariant meaning emerged from within the cultural context of the women. The essential structure of the women's lived experience was one of "wishing for a perfect baby in an altered mode of being while striving for family communion" (Bondas & Eriksson 2001:835). On a superficial level these first two studies appear to have very different findings, but it is important to be aware that Bondas and Eriksson were only considering pregnancy, whereas Barclay et al were exploring pregnancy, birth and the early days post birth. Both indicate that this is a time of some anxiety for the women.

Using content analysis of focus groups and interviews, Cronin (2003) also explored motherhood. The key themes seem to have little relationship with those found by Bondas and Eriksson (2001). An exception to this, though, is their theme of 'altered mode of being' and, like Bondas and Eriksson (2001), she highlights the significance of family. The differences may be in part due to Cronin's study having a focus on need, whereas Bondas and Eriksson's study was more open.

There were four concepts in Cronin's study (2003); birth and hospitalisation, support, motherhood and psychological issues. Within each of these there were a number of key themes found. The major findings seem to be very similar to those of Barclay et al (1997), despite being undertaken on different sides of the world. Given that both Cronin and Barclay et al conducted their studies after the women had become mothers and been through the process of pregnancy, birth and the early days afterwards, it is less surprising that the findings are more similar to each other than with those of Bondas and Eriksson (2001). The women in Cronin's study

(2003) found that coping with the lifestyle changes was difficult, but that they gradually adapted to their new roles, as did those in Barclay et al's study (1997) and Miller's study (2007).

The study, undertaken by Miller (2007), used a longitudinal narrative approach through interview data. Three interviews were conducted with each participant: one prior to the birth (approximately 8 months pregnant), the second after the six-week postnatal check and the third when the baby was approximately eight months old.

This narrative approach led to a discursive paper exploring the experiences of the women (Miller 2007). In their transition to motherhood, the women, in the beginning, try to do the right thing and be responsible, which is similar to the women in Bondas and Eriksson's (2001) study. Initially, they appear to trust the official political discourses of motherhood that birth and mothering will come naturally to them and, if they should have problems, that medicine will address these. Although these discourses were not highlighted in the previous studies, Miller suggests these are social discourses of our society. The women held the belief that they would remain in control of their bodies and confidently know what they were doing. From this starting point the women's experiences of birth were not what they expected and they felt let down by both their own bodies and the professionals.

During the birth of their babies the women experienced loss of control and felt as though they were failures. Eventually, the women gained confidence in their ability to mother and developed relationships with their babies. These findings during and after the birth closely resemble those of Barclay et al's (1997) main findings and are similar to those of Cronin (2003), except they are couched in different terms, probably due to differing methodological approaches.

Cronin's study (2003) is much more pragmatic than the more interpretative study conducted by Miller (2007) or the descriptive study of Bondas and Eriksson (2001). Her focus was on the needs, perceptions and experiences of first-time mothers. As with Barclay et al (1997) and Miller (2007) she found that the new mothers experienced shock, but for Cronin (2003) and Miller (2007) this was primarily due to the birth experience, whereas for Barclay et al (1997) it was the realisation of what motherhood entailed.

Barclay et al (1997) and Miller's (2007) studies may appear to be a rather negative view of motherhood, in comparison to Bondas and Eriksson (2001). This is, perhaps, unsurprising since Bondas and Eriksson's participants were looking forward, with some anxiety, to the event, whereas the others were considering the event in retrospect. However, many of the struggles and concerns for the women are similar for all the studies considered above. Despite some of this negativity, they all suggest women eventually work things out and are able to mother their babies. Perhaps the most significant difference in the studies is that Bondas and Eriksson's study has family communion as a significant feature.

For all the women in the studies of Bondas and Eriksson, Barclay et al, Cronin and Miller, motherhood involved quite monumental changes in all areas of their lives. After an unspecified time they appeared to adjust to these and to strive to become what has been labelled 'good mothers'.

Given that motherhood can be accepted as both becoming and being a mother and the literature seems to suggest that women at this time strive to become a 'good mother' (Brown et al. 1997, Bondas and Eriksson 2001, Marchant 2004, Magill-Cuerden 2006, Miller 2007), it is important that this concept is explored and understood. The next section will, therefore, explore the literature to gain an understanding of what it means to be a good mother.

To be a 'Good Mother'

> "the 'good mother' is required to be loving and caring, to have 'never ending' supplies of patience.....remain calm and relaxed at all times...good listener and communicator...sensitive to children's' needs" *(Brown et al 1997:5).*

Popular online magazines, such as Parenting, inform us that to be a good mother the woman needs to be "adaptable, patient, loving, compassionate, empathetic, kind, strong and determined" (Suttie-Gunson 2007:1). Suttie-Gunson (2007) goes on to say that a good mother will sacrifice anything for her children, that she loves them unconditionally, and forgives them any pain they cause. This is followed up with the advice to 'follow your instincts and you will be a good mother'. This is in contrast to a number of studies that suggest it takes time for women to reach an intuitive responding to their babies (Barclay et al 1996, Cronin 2003, Wilkins 2006, Miller 2007).

There are many cultural images of motherhood and mothers like those above, from media images to early childhood fairy tales of romantic love and 'happy ever after' marriage and motherhood. "Society tells us that motherhood is natural and blissful. The beautiful Madonna adorns church frescos. Smiling, sun-kissed supermodels hold their babies in a modern mimicry of this ancient motif." (Stewart 2004:107).

Whilst most would recognise these as idealised images, feminists inform us that women have internalised these images and carry a vision of the perfect mother into their journey to motherhood (Stewart 2004). Whether the extreme view offered by feminists is accurate or not, conversations with those becoming mothers inform us that there is a sense of the 'good mother' that they are trying to achieve (Miller 2007).

Brown et al (1997) explored the concept of 'good mother', considering whether there were significant changes to this over the recent decades, given the social and cultural changes. They also explored if those women who became depressed during early motherhood did, indeed, have a more unrealistic view of motherhood than those who did not develop depression; a commonly held belief. To do this they initially conducted a survey of recent mothers, including an assessment using the Edinburgh Post Natal Depression Scale (EPNDS). They then did a follow up study, again sending out questionnaires including the EPNDS. Once these were completed, each respondent was interviewed using semi-structured interviewing.

They considered if, as had been suggested, there were two differing discourses of the 'good mother': the original 'good mother' being the stereotype prior to recent, but huge, societal changes and the new 'good mother' as the stereotype after these changes. The old or original 'good mother' was identified as being a woman who focused on love and security for her child and with other passive attributes, such as patience and reliability. The new 'good mother' was said to be interested in her own independence and individuality: she focused on providing stimulation for her child's development.

Despite the identified new stereotype of a 'good mother', all the women (Brown et al 1997) accepted a stereotype most like the traditional view of a 'good mother'. That is, they believed a mother should primarily be loving and caring, with never-ending patience. The mother should be calm and relaxed at all times, be a good communicator, and be understanding and sensitive to the needs of the child. Instead of leaving this stereotype, to associate themselves with a new stereotype of modern mothers who were independent and stimulating, they seemed to have included the stimulation and guidance in the original stereotype.

Unlike predictions of a change of stereotype to correspond with societal change where more women are in professional and full-time paid employment, the women (Brown et al 1997) assimilated new ideas into an existing concept. Piaget (Barker 2007) might suggest the new stereotype was not distinct or different enough to cause cognitive dissonance or unbalance their equilibrium and lead to accommodation of a new schema or stereotype. The women had assimilated new thoughts into an old schema, in this case the stereotype of a 'good mother'.

Despite a generally accepted belief that women who suffer from postnatal depression after the birth of their baby have significantly more unrealistic expectations of motherhood, there was no difference between those with depression and those without. Both the women who scored highly on the EPNDS and the women who did not, held the same stereotype of a 'good mother' (Brown et al 1997).

This stereotype of the 'good mother' seems to be pervasive and enduring, with Campbell in a Christian text in 1984 saying that mother love is different to other sorts of love. He describes it as maternal tenderness, the mother as comforter, interpreter and as a warm presence in a frightening world. Marchant (2004), twenty years later in a recent midwifery text, offers a similar description of the 'good mother'. She states that mothering is altruistic caring, undemanding and selfless love.

This type of motherhood and the stereotype of 'good mother' is, though, culturally determined and influenced by the cultural hegemony. Prior to the eighteenth century children were seen mostly as economic resources and by some even despised as little animals. The industrial revolution and protestant evangelism have probably been the most influential factors in the current stereotype (Muniz 2008). Scientific motherhood in the nineteenth century, which can be viewed alongside the professional and paternalistic ideologies, probably gave rise to the current 'good mother' stereotype. The scientific motherhood only recognised those mothers who were able to devote their time fully to their babies and children as good mothers. Women who needed to do paid employment did not count as true mothers.

A 'good mother' is totally, loving, caring, patient, kind, selfless, sensitive, understanding and so much more, according the stereotypes held by women, told in stories and text books and promoted in the media. To add to this, I would suggest, unachievable way of being, there is also the pressure of the baby or child being damaged without it; "Everything depends on the mother" (Russell cited Exley 2004).

Summary

This chapter has explored what motherhood is, the experiences of women becoming mothers and the expectations of mothers, including those expectations which they put on themselves (Brown et al 1997).

The transition to motherhood is the process of becoming a mother through pregnancy, birth and the early days after the birth, as it takes women a little time after the birth to adjust and become a mother (Barclay et al 1996, Cronin 2003, Wilkins 2006).

There is general agreement that, within the cultural hegemony, there are social expectations of mothers – those who experience motherhood (Marchant 2004, Magill-Cuerden 2006, Miller 2007). Motherhood is enacted within a social and political arena, which influences the dominant discourses on mothering (Littlewood and McHugh 1997, Rothman 2000, Magill-Cuerden 2006, Miller 2007). With monumental changes occurring for the women (Barclay et al 1996, Bondas and Eriksson 2001, Cronin 2003, Miller 2007) and cultural pressures influenced by the dominant discourses of medicine and nature (Miller 2007), women strive to be 'good mothers' (Brown et al 1997, Bondas and Eriksson 2001, Marchant 2004, Magill-Cuerden 2006, Miller 2007). The 'good mother' appears to be an unachievable, generally-held stereotype.

A mother is:

> "she is their earth…
> she is their food and their bed and the extra blanket
> when it grows cold in the night; she is their warmth and their health and their shelter"
> (Hathaway cited Exley 2004)

CHAPTER TWO

WHO SUPPORTS WOMEN BECOMING MOTHERS?

Introduction

There are a number of sources from which women might seek and/ or receive support in becoming a mother. This chapter will briefly consider the support needs of women at this time, what support is and who might be able to provide support for them. This will include a consideration of the role of the baby's father, nurses, doulas (those people, usually women, who offer a social and emotional presence to women during the birth) and midwives.

Support

Morrison and Bennett (2006: 361) clearly state that "we all need support". The National Service Framework (NSF) for children, young people and maternity services in England (DoH 2004) likewise states that women should be 'supported' during pregnancy, birth and in the care of themselves and their babies after birth. They also state that, as part of this support, women should be 'encouraged' to have as 'normal' a pregnancy and birth as possible. For both midwifery and obstetrics, care should be based on good outcomes, clinically and psychologically, whilst putting equal emphasis on preparation for parenthood (DoH 2004). Provision of care and preparation for parenthood could both be seen to be supportive activities. Support can also be seen to underlie the National Institute for Clinical Excellence antenatal (NICE 2003) and postnatal care (NICE 2006) guidelines, with their focus on women-centred care and informed decision making. If, as is suggested, we all need support and that a core concept within midwifery and obstetric care is support, there is a need to clarify what support is and why it is important, prior to exploring who supports women on their journey to motherhood.

Support v.t.n.

A dictionary definition of support is:

1. Carry, hold up, keep from falling or sinking
2. enable to last out, keep from failing, give strength to, encourage
3. endure, tolerate
4. supply with necessities, provide for
5. lend assistance or countenance to, back up, second, further
6. hear out, tend to substantiate or corroborate, bring facts to confirm
7. keep up or represent adequately (Sykes 1982:1072)

The dictionary definition, as demonstrated above, does not offer a precise understanding of support; it provides a number of options, not all of which are listed here. With other words it is clear which meaning is appropriate in a given context, for the word 'support' this is not the case. All of the above definitions could apply to the context of offering support to women on their journey to motherhood. It would, though, appear prudent at this point to distinguish between physical and social support. The support advocated by Morrison and Bennett (2006), that they suggest we all need, might be considered to be social support. Physical support, although having some blurred edges to its definition, can be seen to link more closely to the first dictionary definition of carry, hold up, keep from falling.

Social support appears a rather more flexible concept and can be defined as the resources provided by one person to enhance the well-being of the other (McCourt 2003) but this is so broad that it offers little understanding of the support needed and given to women in their transition to motherhood. It is also worth acknowledging that social support can include physical activities, although it is probably more helpful to label these mostly as practical activities in this situation. To develop a clearer understanding of social support, it may be useful to explore what it does and what it looks like.

Social support is said to have an enormous influence on health and well-being, which has led to a number of theories being developed to understand the phenomenon. Psychologists have developed theories, such as the direct effect and the stress buffer theory, where the social support provides a buffer against the impact of stress on health (Morrison and Bennett 2006). It is likely that these psychological theories underpin the sociological theories (McCourt 2003). Sociological theories, such as 'support can be a protective factor against illness' are widely accepted, but evidence to support them, though, is limited (Morrison and Bennett 2006). Other sociological theories suggest that support can facilitate recovery from illness and is protective against psychosocial risk factors. The research evidence to support these theories arises from sociology, psychology and physiological research, which demonstrate a positive impact of support on health (McCourt 2003).

Lazarus and Folkman (1984) recognise the positive effect of social support in their cognitive, phenomenological appraisal model of stress. Within this, social support can be seen as a coping resource, but it may also affect the primary appraisal of a given situation. Their model can offer, to those interested in this area, a mechanism for understanding the interaction between the impact of stress and social support.

It is useful to consider here the relationship between social support and stress, as the journey to motherhood is recognised as a stressful one (Diemer 1997). Using Lazarus and Folkman's (1991) model, which involves primary appraisal, secondary appraisal, responses and coping can facilitate an understanding of social support's influence on a woman's health and well-being through its mediating effect on stress.

The first stage in their model is primary appraisal; this is where a situation is identified by the individual as positive, negative or neutral. Social support could influence this primary appraisal or perception of a situation. A negative primary appraisal could lead to a stress response. When, for example, a woman is attending for an ultrasound scan, she could primarily appraise this as a negative situation. She may think she needs the scan because the doctor or midwife believes there is something wrong with her or her baby, as people normally have scans to facilitate diagnosis of disorder. A positive primary appraisal could be that a scan will give her the opportunity to see how well her baby is doing. Social support could influence how the scan is perceived and therefore influence whether the woman goes on to experience a stress response. Social support in this situation could involve a wide variety of experiences, such as the woman's partner being excited about the scan as they would like to see the baby, or being given information about the scan and why it is being undertaken.

Secondary appraisal occurs for the woman when she considers her resources to manage a situation. In this appraisal, social support could offer her the resources she needs. Social support at this stage could include her partner attending the scan with her to advocate for her. If the woman appraises the situation, such as the scan, as negative and she does not have the resources to manage the situation, she may then develop stress responses which could be physiological, psychological or social. Lazarus and Folkman (1991) suggest that this may not be a purely linear process and there may be a going back and forth between stages.

Once the person, in this case a woman, perceives stress she will, most likely, attempt to develop coping strategies to manage or eliminate the stress response. These coping strategies can be adaptive or maladaptive, helpful or unhelpful for the person's ongoing health and wellbeing. Adaptive coping responses can be further divided into problem solving and emotional strategies. Social support could either assist in resolving the problem situation, problem solving, or facilitate emotional coping.

To return to the example, if the women perceives undergoing a scan as negative and does not perceive herself to have sufficient resources to influence or control the situation, she may experience a stress response. This could include physical (e.g. shaking, sweating, vomiting, light-headedness), psychological (e.g. reduced attention, concentration, memory) and social elements (e.g. irritability with others, lack of responsiveness and sensitivity to others). The stress response is uncomfortable for people and they, therefore, look for ways of ameliorating the experience. For this woman she may chose not to attend the scan, which is one way of solving the problem of the stress response, but this type of avoidance behaviour is considered maladaptive. There are a myriad of other ways in which she might attempt to cope, including crying (emotion-focused and for short periods can be adaptive), seeking support from others (usually considered a problem-solving approach and adaptive), or drinking alcohol (emotion-focused and maladaptive).

When an example, as given above, is considered using the Lazarus and Folkman cognitive phenomenological interactive appraisal model (1991) it is easy to recognise how social support can be of benefit. At all stages of the model, some type of social support can prevent the occurrence of a stress response, ameliorate or reduce it.

There do not appear to be any studies conducted to assess whether social support facilitates the woman's appraisal of whether she has achieved being a 'good mother', as described in the previous chapter. The Lazarus and Folkman model of stress offers a constructive view of stress management and the significant role social support can play. The model would uphold an example of women in the secondary appraisal stage assessing their resources to be sufficient to be a 'good mother' and hence not experiencing unpleasant stress responses or with support in the primary appraisal stage not perceiving their lack of being the stereotypical 'good mother' as negative.

McCourt (2003) suggests that social support can be divided into emotional, informational and practical support. Others include esteem support (Ogden 2000, Mander 2001) but Morrison and Bennett (2006) go on to identify network support as well. Mander (2001) warns that to pay too great attention to the divisions between different types of social support is not always helpful. Despite this, these divisions can be useful as they offer some flexibility to allow for individual differences and needs, including culture. In the context of understanding the support needed and experienced by women becoming mothers, they facilitate further examination.

Emotional support and practical social support are generally perceived to be quite different and easily distinguished. Practical support could involve someone helping with child-care, cooking, shopping etc. for the woman, whereas emotional support is usually seen more in terms of listening, showing concern and intimacy (Mander 2001). Informational support for women might include the providing of leaflets, giving talks or showing the woman around the birthing unit. To be supportive, this information-giving needs to be associated with giving the right information at the right time to facilitate reduced stress.

Esteem support can be seen to be similar to emotional support and that is probably why some texts only identify emotional support. Esteem support is identified as different from emotional support when it occurs in relation to the woman feeling vulnerable or at risk. The supporter in this situation offers encouragement and facilitates the woman's belief in herself; it can also be undertaken in the same manner as emotional support, by listening and showing concern. Network support is believed to offer a sense of belonging and affiliation (Morrison and Bennett 2006). For the woman becoming a mother, feeling part of a group, whether that is friends, family or parent-craft groups, can be seen as network support.

It is likely that women need different amounts and types of support at different times. This can also involve various people at differing moments and, perhaps, in each type of support. For example, a mother might provide emotional support, a teacher might supply informational support and a cleaner might provide practical support. All of the writers identified above also accept that support can be actual or perceived and suggest it is the perception of support that is most significant for women.

The sources of social support are usually divided into two categories: informal or unpaid and formal or paid (McCourt 2003). Those that usually fall into the informal category are partners, family and other relatives, friends and neighbours. Formal social support for women in transition to motherhood can include their General Practitioner (GP / family doctor), Midwife (maternity nurse), Obstetrician, Social Worker, Health Visitor, Mental Health Nurse, Psychiatrist, Doula. The support provided by the family (including partner or father of the baby) is of paramount importance for women on their journey to motherhood, but the support given by others can still have an impact on the woman's emotional well-being (Ball 1994).

Each of these supporters, both formal and informal, can assist in the woman's journey to motherhood. For some women the experience is one of being supported by each of the above in different ways. For other women, the majority of their social support is provided by informal carers; partner, family and friends. There are some women, though, who have limited social networks and need to fulfil their support needs through formal services.

Informal Social Support

Fathers

The role of fathers has changed over recent years; in the past it has been assumed he would provide certain limited types of support for the woman and baby, such as financial support. In Western society there is now the expectation that the father will take part in prenatal education classes, attend the birth and support mother and baby after the birth. It is becoming increasingly recognised, though, alongside their supporting role, that fathers need to develop their own relationship with their infants (Mander 2001). The father can, therefore, be seen to have a duality of role and it may be that fathers, along with mothers, need informative, emotional and practical support.

Fathers are seen as the primary source of social support for most women on their journey to motherhood (Sarestano et al 1999, Gee et al 2007). Social support offered by them has been shown to mitigate some of the impact of the stress experienced on the transition to motherhood. He is said to be unique and irreplaceable (Sarestano et al 1999). The social support offered by fathers has been generally considered to be influenced by ethnicity (Gee et al 2007) but the father's support has been found to be more significantly influenced by age and marital status (Sarestano et al 1999).

Sarestano et al (1999) were particularly interested in the extent to which ethnicity, within the United States of America (USA), influenced social support for women during pregnancy. Previous literature had suggested there were large differences according to the ethnic background of the mothers-to-be. Social support, as has already been stated, has been found to improve outcomes for mother and baby. In this large study they found that, whilst ethnicity is influential in the provision of social support, this type of support received from the baby's father was mostly influenced by marital status, but age was also significant. If the father was married to the woman becoming a mother, the woman reported a higher level of support. Also, younger women usually perceived themselves to receive more support from the fathers of their babies than older women.

In measuring social support by fathers, various scales have been used in research, such as the eight item perceived support scales by Turner et al (1983, 1990) which was used by Sarestano et al (1999). This included the extent to which the father was affectionate, understood feelings, talked to and spent time with the mother, was dependable financially and was willing to help with the baby. The received 12 item social support scale Sarestano et al (1999) used was described by Collins et al (1993) and included material support provided, assistance with tasks, advice or information and the father's involvement by listening. Diemer, (1997) when considering the social support of fathers, accepted that it involved helping with housework, coping by seeking social support and seeking information from the woman's doctor. These scales and activities were used to measure the social support offered by the fathers.

Young mothers, supported by their spouse or partner in the manner identified above, experienced reduced psychological distress, higher self-esteem and more overall life satisfaction (Gee et al 2007). For first-time mothers, the perceived emotional support from fathers has been found to reduce the risk of psychological distress and post-natal depression (Cappuccini & Cochrane 2000). Where fathers are involved in supporting the women, the outcomes are good for the women so they, and those caring for them, should encourage the involvement of fathers (Mander 2001).

The expectation of the father to support women through the whole journey to motherhood, through pregnancy, birth and post-natal, with limited social support (information, emotional, practical) themselves, may offer one explanation for the disillusionment of some women (Mander 2001). Men have been reported to feel uncomfortable in the labouring room of the woman, due to her expectations for intense emotional support when his expectations were to offer coaching on tasks such as 'breathing through the pain'. This may be due to the parent-craft classes attended prior to the birth, with their focus on the physical elements of the experience. There is also evidence that women, despite expressing the desire for help with the baby, ignore the fathers input, thereby confirming their belief that they are unsupported. This then could become a self-fulfilling prophesy, with fathers not trying to help in case it is ignored (Mander 2001).

It is suggested that women actively seek the father's help and not assume they will need to do all the tasks. This should facilitate the support of each other and enhance the relationship as, within this type of committed relationship, the father is more able to socially support the woman (Sarestano et al 1999).

It has been contested that the father should be seen by the midwife as the 'third patient' after the woman and baby. Patient is not usually a term preferred by midwives, as women are not generally 'ill' when pregnant and giving birth. It is also probably impracticable for the midwife to see the father as the third patient as, when a woman is birthing, she will probably need the entire of the midwife's attention.

Fathers are said to need education and support to be able to support women, as it is also a transition for them and their paternal role models may encourage them into traditional, gender-based roles, rather than the more egalitarian role that may be expected by the women (Diemer 1997). Gender-based conditioning can influence the man's desire and ability to show concern and seek support for themselves or their partners. The stereotype of the strong, decisive man in control, may force the father to play down his feeling of helplessness and weakness, thus making him unavailable for the support women need (Schott 2005). Where the father's role-model is his own father (baby's grandfather) and he (baby's grandfather) has a traditional gender-based role, when the father takes an egalitarian role the couple (baby's mother and father) are at higher risk of marital disharmony (Diemer 1997). Fletcher (2009) offers an insightful approach to promoting infant and mother well-being by supporting the father.

Fletcher (2009) focused on the father infant interactions to facilitate the well-being of the baby when the mother experiences post-natal depression. He found that, by focusing on promoting the father-baby bond and developing this relationship, not only was the father and baby's well-being enhanced, but also the mother's. In this paper he only offers one case study, but it should be useful for further thought, research and intervention. There are others, such as Schott (2005), who identify the need for parent education, focused on informing men and providing them with alternative role models and peer support.

It is clear that the father has an important part to play in the support of women becoming mothers, but it is also important not to lose sight of the father's needs. The relationships between mother and father and between parents and baby are crucial for the well-being of each of them. So, although the father is needed to provide social support for women becoming mothers, it is essential that they are cared for too.

Family and Friends

Social networks, such as the family (including the baby's father), friends and neighbours can be seen to be the primary source of social support for women on their journey to motherhood (McCourt 2003). It is therefore important that they are considered here. "Families are said to be the building blocks and they remain the basic unit for the protection and rearing of young children. They provide emotional and financial support for both adults and children" (Dunn-Toroosian 2003: 69).

The family can be seen to be culturally-determined from most sociological perspectives, but what constitutes a family is contentious within contemporary literature. Politically, in the UK, there appears to be an identification of the family as one man, one woman and their children (the nuclear family). This is despite the diverse nature of families in western society, with some families extended (the extended family) with grandparents, aunts and uncles, cousins etc. and other families with only one adult or same sex couples with children. Western society appears to hold a number of differing cultural groups which determine the nature of a family, but political agendas and associated legislation are not always organised to support this diversity.

Within the family, as with all social groups, there are expectations about the roles each member will play (Hogg and Vaughan 1998). It has been recognised that social support from family and friends is strongly linked to ethnicity (Sarestano et al 1999). Within the USA, African-American women report more support from their families than Latinas and white women. African-American and Latinas women all identify the quality of support from their families as higher than the white American women. White American women indicated that they have larger friendship groups and receive more support from them than the other two groups of women. This can be seen to be linked to their cultural backgrounds, the culture in which they grew up and the amount of time the ethnic group has been part of the USA.

Sarestano et al (1999) explored social support from families using six item questionnaires, which included whether the woman's family were there if needed, if the woman could rely on the family, whether they thought she was a worthwhile person, had confidence in her, would help her with problems and would stand by her. For the African-American women and the white women, there appears to be an expectation that they will strive for independence. Despite this, if the African- American women needed support there was the expectation that the family would provide it. For the white American women, their strong individualistic culture appears to lead them to develop large friendship networks outside of the family. This culture appears to lead them to gain support, initially from their partner and then from friends. It is suggested that Latino women live within a culture of 'familism' with the expectation that social support will be provided by the extended family.

The ethnic differences identified did appear to influence the amount and quality of the perceived support the women received from family and friends. White women reported the highest amount of support, but this was primarily from the baby's father, whereas the African-Americans and Latino women reported higher levels of support from family and friends (Sarestano et al 1999). Sarestano et al (1999) warn us, though, that this is a complex area and support from family and friends is influenced by a number of factors, including ethnicity, social economic standing, age, parity and marital status.

Women who have a greater sense of well-being tend to rate their social support as high (McCourt 2003), but for researchers this can create the dilemma of 'is their well- being high because their social support from family and friends is high' or 'do they rate the support highly because they have a high sense of well-being'.

Social support from family and friends would appear to be important for the woman's well-being on her journey to motherhood, but to assume that this is the area the women will receive the support they need is risky. As has been seen for some women, their support needs can be, and are, met by family, but for others this is not the case and, whilst ethnicity may indicate the likelihood of the women receiving sufficient support from her family, this should not be stated as the rule.

Voluntary agencies and organisations

There are numerous voluntary, charitable agencies and organisations that offer support to those becoming a mother. Perhaps the most well known in the UK is the National Childbirth Trust, who offer support via the world wide web, nationally and locally. They provide information, education and social support groups both prior to the birth of a baby and after the birth. Thousands of women in the UK access their facilities each year through becoming a member. For parents who are in receipt of social financial support the current fee is two pounds per year (2010 NCT). On their website many women express how helpful their support has been. The development of the world wide web has seen a proliferation of support available via home computers with organisations such as netmums and facebook. Other more focused support groups have been accessible for women for a number of years but they too offer information and support through their websites. Examples are the La Leche League who promote and support breastfeeding and the Marce society whose focus is on mental health through pregnancy, childbirth and early motherhood.

It is difficult to assess how many women use the support available from these sources as most can be accessed anywhere in the world except where membership of the organisation is necessary. The availability of the world wide web has meant that women can access information they want when they want it but social contact can still be limited by their geographical location. Accessing information from websites may be difficult for people whose first language is not widely spoken or where they have language difficulties for a variety of other reasons. Certainly the women described by the midwives in my study did not appear to be knowledgeable about the support available to them and needed to be guided by the midwives.

Formal Social Support

Family Doctors / General Practitioners (GP)

Most people within the UK are registered with a General Practitioner, who some people still refer to as their family doctor. There are some groups within society that are not registered, for example people in prisons, although, more recently, this group of people has been offered care through the Primary Care Trusts (PCTs), as with most of the general population in the UK. Despite this, the organisation of health services in the UK is being restructured, so care provision will soon change again. Health and social care provision in the UK and the USA are 'hot' political topics that generate much discussion and dissent. Groups such as the homeless, Gypsy and Traveller groups, in the UK, are not usually registered with a General Practitioner, but they can access emergency health care through accident and emergency units. The formal social support, from health services, of women becoming mothers within these groups is more difficult to access and varies between geographical areas.

General Practitioners in the UK are the gatekeepers to formal National Health Service (NHS) care (RCGP 2010). Women usually attend their GP when they believe they are pregnant, or are attempting to conceive, and once pregnancy is confirmed, the GP will put them in contact with the midwife attached to their General Practice surgery. Some women choose to access independent midwives, but this is not paid for by the NHS, it is private (paid for over and above the taxes paid to fund the NHS) care.

The GP 'gate-keeps', gives access to, the provision for the whole healthcare needs of the woman and baby, prior to, throughout pregnancy and post birth, but the midwives and obstetricians plan, implement and evaluate the care associated with pregnancy, birth and the early days after the birth. Midwives liaise with GPs if they assess the women to need specialist care, such as mental health services, to facilitate access to them.

Family doctors or GPs can be seen to be the people who can provide access to formal social support for the majority of women in the UK. The GP may provide social support themselves, as they listen (emotional support) to their patients with compassion and respect (esteem support) and provide the information (information support) and resources (practical support) that are perceived necessary.

It can be seen that GPs play an important role in the provision of social support for women on their journey to motherhood, but it is very time-limited, appointments usually last only ten minutes. Some GPs play a more extensive role and attend home births and maternity unit births, but all births are attended by midwives and some solely by them.

Nurses

Within the UK there are four fields of nursing and there are specialisms in each of these. In the NHS, alongside the four fields of nursing; adult, mental health, child and learning disability, there are associated professions, such as midwives. The structure of the NHS provides care for women becoming mothers, through midwifery services or midwives.

In other countries the organisation of care for these women is different. Most states in the USA have maternity nurses who care for women during the birthing process, under the supervision of obstetricians, and public health nurses provide care after the birth. In Finland the care is very similar, with public health nurses providing the pre- natal and post-natal care and maternity nurses / midwives supporting women through the birth (Kuosmanen 2010).

The role of midwives and maternity nurses in providing social support of women on their journey to motherhood will be considered later in this chapter; this section is focusing on the support offered by the four fields of nursing identified above.

Adult Nursing

Adult nurses work with people over sixteen years of age, although this is not a strictly applied division and there is sometimes a need for them to support people who are younger, particularly in certain specialist areas. Their focus is on the physical health needs of people, although, as with the other fields of nursing, they are expected to provide holistic care, assessing for and ensuing care provision for all the health and social care needs of the people with whom they work. This may be undertaken by providing nursing care alongside other health and social care practitioners (NHS 2010). Within this field there are a number of specialisms. These specialisms generally are in line with those of medicine, such as ophthalmic or surgery, but some are specific to adult nursing, for example continence nurses.

Whilst it is generally the midwife that coordinates the care of a woman becoming a mother, other adult nursing specialists may be involved. For example if a woman is pregnant but also has a physical health problem of diabetes, the diabetic nurse (from the adult field of nursing) may also be involved in her care. These specialist nurses will usually offer informational or practical social support.

Child Nursing

A children's nurse may offer social support to women, but this is normally after the baby has been born. If the baby has physical health problems or is premature, a child nurse may have responsibility for their physical care needs and may support the woman with this. They can offer support with other child health needs, such as feeding and sleeping behaviours. Despite this, they are not generally involved with newborn babies unless there is a particular physical health problem, such as babies born with a heart problem.

If a child nurse needs to be involved in the woman's journey to motherhood it will be through the needs of her baby, but they may offer any support needs the mother may have, except for her physical health. They could offer informational and practical support in regard to her baby. They would assess her social and financial support needs and provide her with information to address these, perhaps with the assistance of a social worker. A focus of children's nurses is to support the mother and other family members so that they can undertake the baby's care and this may mean, for example, offering guidance and encouragement to bond with the baby.

Child nurses may offer the woman all the types of support needs identified earlier, such as emotional (listening to her concerns), esteem (encouraging her interactions with her baby), networking (putting her in touch with other parents who have similar experiences) and practical (undertaking the physical care tasks she is unable to do).

Although child nurses may offer all types of social support, for most women they do not need the involvement of a child nurse as they only have contact with them if there is a health problem with the baby. The majority of women do not have contact with, or receive support from, child nurses as their baby does not have health problems and if they did, it would only account for one part of their journey to motherhood.

Learning Disability Nursing

Women with a learning disability may become mothers, as with many other women with disabilities, and they may be supported by a learning disability nurse alongside regular care from GPs and midwives. The main role of a learning disability nurse is to ensure that people with these disabilities gain the opportunities, respect and care they require. Learning disability nurses aim to facilitate people achieving their potential and living as independently as possible (NHS careers 2010).

The Valuing People Now (DH 2009) document sets out the vision that people with learning disabilities have the right to lead their lives as they choose and have the same opportunities and responsibilities as other members of society. In accordance with this, the governmental White Paper, Equity and Excellence; liberating the NHS (DH 2010), states that people, regardless of disability or cultural group, should have equal rights to health care.

The focus of learning disability nurses is to ensure that people with these conditions can manage their own lives in an environment free from discrimination. If a woman with a learning disability were to become pregnant, she would only need their support if her learning disability interfered with her ability to access appropriate care and support. It may be that she would not need to access support from one of these nurses.

If the woman was being supported by a learning disability nurse prior to becoming pregnant, they would support her through the whole journey and afterwards as a mother if she continued to need this. They may also be asked to be part of the care provided by midwifery services to support the midwife and or the woman over this period, as it is stressful for the woman and learning disability nurses have knowledge and skills that might help the midwife. The support they can offer is wide ranging and can included all the areas of social support already identified for both woman with a learning disability and her carers, whether they are formal or informal (DH 2007).

Mental health Nursing

The focus of mental health nursing can be seen to be helping or caring for those with mental health problems. This becomes problematic, as mental health can fluctuate more rapidly than physical health. As with other areas of nursing there is also the expectation that mental health nurses will become involved in health promotion; they are expected to promote mental health.

Within midwifery, as will be seen throughout this book, there has been considered to be a duality of approach which has also been recognised in mental health nursing. This dichotomy of the philosophy of care has been labelled as art and science. This is not unique within nursing, it can be found in most practice-based disciplines (Norman and Ryrie 2009).

The underpinning philosophy of art and science appear to be a tension within both nursing and midwifery, but the conflicting approaches appear to more problematic for midwives. The concerns over this dichotomy in mental health nursing have reduced recently, as the profession can be seen to be forming a consensual approach to the use of interpersonal (artistic) and the evidence-based care (science) (Norman and Ryrie 2009). Mental health nurses acknowledge the essential need to develop relationships with their clients (artistic). Whilst tried and tested interventions (science) are accepted as useful, there is still the desire to look for new ways of working to facilitate those with mental health problems gaining a greater quality of life. Therefore, mental health nurses primarily develop relationships with people with mental health issues and facilitate their overcoming these to live independent and fulfilling lives.

Mental health nurses work with people throughout their lifespan. This means that they could be working with a woman throughout her journey to motherhood if she had mental health problems. There are also mental health nurses who specialise in maternal mental health. As with learning disability nurses, their role could also be to offer support to midwives in their care of women at this time. The transition to motherhood is a stressful time (Diemer 1997) and many women struggle with their mental health during pregnancy and the early days after the birth.

The majority of women experience some emotional lability which is usually labelled the 'baby blues' (around 50 – 80% of women) (Evins and Theofastous1997). Although the incident rates for depression is suggested to be 10% (Lawrie et al 2002) Gavin et al (2005) offer incident rates of 12.9% prenatally and 19.2% postnatal, with post-partum psychosis affecting less than 1% (Evins and Theofastous1997). There can therefore be seen to be a large number of women who may benefit from the support of mental health nurses. This is not a new phenomenon. Greaves (2009) found evidence for post natal depression in ancient Greece, some two and a half thousand years ago.

Mental health nurses and psychiatrists are said to be the main collaborators when treating women with mental illness after the birth of their babies (Engqvist et al 2010) but those involved in the woman's care extend to other health care professionals: midwives, obstetricians and child health practitioners. It has, though, been found that even brief interventions with a mental health nurse can have significant improvements for the emotional well-being of women experiencing post-natal depression (Kuosmanen et al 2010).

The support offered by mental health nurses is through their development of therapeutic relationships to develop understanding and ensure the provision of the interventions the woman needs. The provision of social support for the woman, and those caring for her, can be part of these interventions. They can provide emotional care by listening and showing concern, practical support by coordinating the services the women needs, informational support by explaining what might be happening to her and what can be offered to help her, esteem support by showing respect for her knowledge and abilities and network support through family work and engaging her with groups.

Although the mental health nurse can offer extensive social support, they do not have contact with all women on their journey to motherhood and, given their limited numbers, they are usually only involved with those women with the greatest mental health needs.

Social Workers

Social work has its roots in addressing social needs, particularly poverty (Jones 2002). A contemporary view of poverty includes poverty of care, consideration, political voice etc., as well as limited financial resources. Social workers work with people, organisations and societies with the aim of improving the quality of life for those experiencing poverty. The reasons for social work within the UK are said to be poverty, social exclusion, family breakdown, child abuse, domestic violence, ill health, physical disability, frailty of old age, mental illness and learning difficulties (Davies 2002:v).

As with mental health and learning disability nurses, social workers may be involved in the support of women becoming mothers but not in a general sense. They would work alongside health practitioners and voluntary organisations depending on the women's and babies' needs. If the woman was at risk in some manner such as financially, physically (through disability or of physical violence), mentally (previous mental health problems or psychological abuse), socially (she has dependants or is in an abusive relationship), environmentally (limited access to services or living conditions are dangerous), a social worker may be involved.

Social workers usually have specialist areas in which they are employed, as do nurses. They may work within specialist mental health services and support women with mental health problems in a similar way to mental health nurses. Another specialist area is child care, within this area they may involved in assessing potential risks to children or babies and organising appropriate care for them. A common reason for a childcare social worker to become involved with a woman with a baby is the baby's failure to 'thrive' (Waterhouse 2002). A concern would probably have been raised with them by a health care professional already involved in their care such as a midwife or health visitor, but members of the public are encouraged to raise their concerns about their neighbours with social services.

The majority of women, though, do not access support from social workers and the focus of this book is those women who experience a 'normal' transition to motherhood. Therefore the social worker, despite fulfilling an important role for some women in their support needs on their journey to motherhood, is not the key provider of emotional support for women becoming mothers.

Doulas

Doulas are formal supporters of women; they are employed by the woman or her family. Doula is a term widely used in the USA for the person who supports a woman in childbirth, despite some concern around whether this is a derogatory term. It is a Greek word that appears to mean female slave (Mander 2001). Doulas are generally considered to be trained companions, usually supporting women labouring, but some are employed after the baby is born to support the new family in the early days after the birth (Klaus et al 2002).

A doula's primary aim would appear to be providing support for the woman, and some have referred to their activities as 'mothering the mother' (Mander 2001). The doula usually meets the woman once or twice in the third trimester of pregnancy, so that she is a known person when the woman goes into labour. She (most doulas are women) then stays with the woman throughout labour, providing a continuous presence (Klaus et al 2002) offering physical comfort, emotional support, information and advocacy (Mander 2001).

The ongoing presence of the doula has been found to have a significant impact on the childbirth experience, reducing the length of labour in the USA, where midwifery care is mostly undertaken by obstetricians and maternity nurses. The research studies, related to use of non-professionals like doulas, is mixed. Klaus et al (2002) make wide-reaching claims for the outcomes of using doulas but Mander's (2001) consideration of the available research studies would guide maternity service providers to think carefully before embarking on using this approach in their services.

It can be seen that, despite some positive research studies in the USA related to the support offered by doulas, very few women in the UK have accessed one; this may be due to the financial implications and the availability of midwives.

This brief overview of the informal and formal social support of women becoming mothers, has shown that the father and other family members have a vital role to play in supporting women. Nurses and doula can also offer social support, but they are not available to all women in this transition. Within the UK, only GPs and midwives are available to offer social support to all women on their journey. When the limitations of the GPs' availability are clarified, it can be seen that midwives are the key carers who take on the role of offering social support. Midwives are involved with women throughout the process of becoming a mother.

Midwives

Midwives have contact with women from the initial booking appointment, early in pregnancy, until the early days after the birth, usually until the baby is between 10 and 28 days old. The Nursing and Midwifery Council (the governing body of midwives in the UK) states that a midwife "will work in partnership with women and their families to give support, care and advice during pregnancy, labour and the postnatal period" (NMC 2009). The midwives' professional bodies (ICM, RCM), as well as government initiatives (NICE 2003, 2006, NSF 2004), guide midwives to work 'in partnership' with women. The role laid out for midwives by this guidance is complex, requiring a wide repertoire of skills.

Midwives are expected to "work in partnership with" women and their families and they therefore need to develop this, through relationships with women and their families. To provide support, care and advice, as stated, midwives need to be technologically and bio-medically knowledgeable (ICM 2006).

The International Confederation of Midwives (ICM), which works with all United Nations agencies and represents 72 nations of the world, produced a definition of the midwife and outlined the preparation that is required for the role (ICM 2006). They also identified key midwifery concepts, such as respecting dignity and advocating for women, the scope of midwifery practice and the midwifery model of care. What is particularly important is the ICM's provision of the essential competencies for basic midwifery practice. These competencies also fulfil the guidance of the NMC code of conduct (NMC 2008). The ICM gives 6 competencies, which are broken down into basic knowledge and skills, additional knowledge and skills, and professional behaviours. The competencies include a sound knowledge-base from all areas that may influence the woman's experiences, from biological to cultural. They state that midwives need knowledge of, and skills in, pre-pregnancy care and family planning, care and counselling during pregnancy, care during labour and birth, postnatal care and care of the newborn (ICM 2006).

Midwives in the UK are also guided, as previously indicated, by a number of governmental papers, notably 'Changing Childbirth', which advocates choice, continuity and control for pregnant women, which they say facilitates women-centred care (Department of Health 1993). These elements, along with the NICE guidelines (2003, 2006) and NSF (DoH 2004), will directly influence what a midwife does and when. It is also important to recognise that these guidelines do not explicitly conflict with the competencies laid out by the ICM.

Accepting the above, midwives should provide women-centred care and information to facilitate women's informed decision-making. They should provide and organise care, manage common symptoms of pregnancy and perform clinical examinations and screening, using evidence-based approaches (NICE 2003). The post-natal care-giver should provide individualised negotiated care; as part of this, timely information, including the signs and symptoms of potentially life-threatening ill-health of mother and baby. They should also promote breast-feeding. Women should be asked about their support needs and coping strategies and be encouraged to tell health-care professionals about their mood, emotional state and behaviour that is outside of their normal pattern (NICE 2006).

Some overarching skills can be seen in the above lists, which are assessment, provision and evaluation of evidence-based interventions (or non-intervention) in negotiation with women, to ensure women-centred, individualised care. To achieve this, midwives need to develop partnership relationships with women, supported by good communication skills, including information-giving and information-receiving ability. Alongside this, they appear to need clinical skills, such as examination and evidence appraisal skills. The vision provided by the NSF (2004), which is supported by the key concepts of the ICM (2006), both of which name midwives to provide this care, would support the need for the above, but also highlights a need to emphasise the care needs of vulnerable and disadvantaged women, encouraging women to have 'normal' births and helping parents prepare for parenthood.

These guidelines are quite extensive and studies have been undertaken to explore whether midwives are fulfilling them and which guidelines are considered by them to be the most important. Butler et al (2008) set out to find which of the competencies outlined above were the most crucial for those completing their midwifery programmes to work as registered midwives. They found, by conducting a qualitative study, that a wide range of midwives felt that the most crucial elements of being a midwife were being a safe practitioner, having the right attitude and being an effective communicator. Being a safe practitioner had three dimensions, which were having a reasonable degree of self-sufficiency, using up-to-date knowledge, and self and professional awareness. To achieve this it was stated that new midwives needed to have 'the right attitude', which was to be caring, kind, compassionate and empathetic. Without good communication skills it was felt that safe practice and the right attitude would be very difficult to demonstrate.

Despite all the above expectations of a midwife, the one concept that could be seen as central and is regularly used to describe what midwives do is *care* (McCourt et al 2000, Stewart 2004, Page and McCandlish 2006). Indeed, the Nursing Midwifery Council (NMC 2008) identifies that the role of midwives and nurses is to provide care.

The central concept within midwifery can be seen to be 'care' (McCourt et al 2000, Stewart 2004, Page and McCandlish 2006) and the midwife-woman relationship has been identified as the central element of this 'care' (Fleming 1998b, Fraser1999, Walsh 1999, Kirkham 2000, Pairman 2000, McCourt 2005, Hunter 2006). Through this care midwives are expected to provide support. Given the lists above of the tasks and abilities expected of midwives, they appear to be expected to provide all types of social support: emotional, practical and informational.

There is limited information on the emotional support given by midwives, but it does appear to be expected as part of the midwives' role. Chapter 3 discusses the literature available in this area. As with learning disability and mental health nurses, midwives offer emotional support through their partnership relationships with women. Within these, midwives spend time listening and demonstrating their care. Developing and maintaining supportive relationships with women can be difficult within the current culture in health (Fraser 1999, Levy 1999c, Kirkham 2000, Kirkham et al 2002a, Stapleton et al 2002a). These relationships appear to be most easily managed when they are reciprocal, so that both midwives and women gain something out of them (Hunter 2006).

There seems to be quite a wide variation of practical support, both type and amount, offered by midwives, depending on the situation the women are in at the time. Sometimes they offer extensive practical support, for example, when the woman is in labour they may give her practical support by allowing her to lean on them or by getting her a drink of water. The majority of the time midwives, as with nurses, appear to seek to facilitate independence in the woman.

Information giving or information support is recognised as an essential part of a midwife's role (NICE 2003, 2006, DoH 2004). There has been a lot of discussion related to whether accurate information is being given. It has been found that this is not always the case (Kirkham et al 2002a, Stapleton et al 2002a). While some suggest that information is being provided in a woman-centred manner as stipulated (Walsh 1999, McCourt 2005), there is also evidence that this may not be happening (Lomax and Robinson 1996).

Despite the limited consensus on what support is needed for women on their journey to motherhood and how it should be provided, women have identified the need for support in a number of areas through their transition (Edwards 2000). Women want supportive midwifery practices, emotional, spiritual and physical support and supportive qualities in their midwives. Supportive qualities appear to include listening, respect, acceptance and being given clear information (Schuiling and Sampselle 1999, Edwards 2000, Morse 2000). It has also been found that women desire choice and control (McCourt 2003).

When women receive social support on their journey through pregnancy they appear to have reduced anxieties, reduced psychological and physical morbidity. In most cases where social support is received, women experience increased satisfaction with their care and communication and an increased sense of control (Elbourne et al 1989 cited McCourt 2003: 198). For women receiving continuous support during labour, they experienced reduced time in labour, reduced need for medication, less operative deliveries and a lower number of babies with a five minute apgar score of less than 7. Some trials also found a greater satisfaction with the birth, increased duration of breast feeding, decrease in perineal trauma and less potential postnatal depression and difficulties with mothering (Hodnett 1999). It is therefore essential that women receive the social support they require.

Given the issues associated with the provision of social support by informal supporters and lack of robustness for the evidence of doulas ensuring support needs are met, the midwife would appear to be the best person to ensure the woman receives the required social support. The midwife's education should prepare her to recognise the woman's needs on her journey and the skills to ensure her support needs are addressed.

Conclusion

Midwives are viewed as being in an excellent position to support the health and well- being of women and their families, due to their extensive contact with women at a time when they not only needed support, but were receptive to the health messages given (McCourt 2003).

Mother of two children Linda Begbie (2004: 23) states " A sceptic might argue that this sort of emphasis on emotional support and the non-medical aspects of pregnancy is all very well, but that it should stay on the periphery of standard care for pregnant women – left instead to doulas, childbirth educators, active birth teachers and self-taught. I disagree. During my two experiences of childbirth, strong feelings – fear panic, nostalgia, excitement, lack of control – were acute, and – crucially – made a big difference to my physical progress".

It is important to note that midwifery literature informs us that professionals are not the main source of social support for women, except in unusual circumstances. Family friends and neighbours are of overwhelming importance in providing necessary social support (McCourt 2003). Despite this, midwives should have the knowledge and skills to recognise when a woman's support needs are not being met and, by their care enacted through the midwife-woman relationship, address these unmet needs.

> "Perhaps it is not simply who provides the support, but the perceived match between the values of each social support provider and those of the expectant father that is important" (Diemer 1997: 290).

CHAPTER THREE

WHAT IS EMOTIONAL CARE?

Introduction

It was established in the previous chapter that midwives are in the best position to offer emotional care to women and their families on their journey to motherhood. To come to a more detailed understanding of what emotional care is for women at this time, it will be useful to initially establish what care is for midwives and women. This chapter will then go on to clarify how emotional care differs from regular midwifery care. Therefore, this chapter will start with an exploration of literature pertaining to care.

Care

Care or caring can be seen to be a rather nebulous term, being applied to both personal attributes and overt behaviours; it can be both noun and verb. Despite this, most people believe they have a sense of what 'to be caring' means; it is only when there is an attempt to develop a clear definition, that addresses all elements of care, that problems occur. This can be seen in The Nursing and Midwifery Council's (2004: 13) leaflet, which provides the code of professional conduct for nurses and midwives; it offers "to provide help or comfort" as a definition of care, whereas theologians, such as Campbell (1984: 6), offer the definition that

> "Consistent professional care is a form of love. It entails a personal commitment by the person offering care which cannot be captured solely in the language of contract"

There are a number of basic and introductory texts that explore the concept of caring. One such text (Richards 1999) suggests that there are a number of factors which influence care, particularly the caring relationship. The factors include elements such as time available, the care setting, needs of caregiver and receiver, support for both and the skills and expertise of the caregiver. The skills and expertise the caregiver should possess are sensitivity, understanding of care needs and an ability to respond to these needs. For the caregiver to be able to respond to the client's care needs they should develop their communication skills, including empathy and self-awareness (Richards 1999). This demonstrates that caring is a complex and skilful task; despite this there seems to be a general assumption that these are skills or attributes that people possess naturally, that do not require learning and do not attract status (Bolton 2000, John & Parson 2006).

Care and caring are identified as the central process in all the helping professions (Morrison 1992). There have been a number of theorists and researchers interested in the phenomenon of caring, including theologians such as Campbell (1984), nurses such as Leininger (1985), and midwives such as McCourt et al (2000).

Theories related to care have developed over the last few decades; in the 1970s Madeline Leininger proposed a cultural theory of care and Jean Watson the theory of human caring. In the 1980s, Simone Roach established her theory of human caring in nursing and in the 1990s Boykin and Schoenhofer their theory of nursing as caring (McCance et al 1999). These theories originated from differing conceptual origins but have similarities, in that they all at least imply that nursing care is humanistic in nature and involves "attitudes and values on the one hand and activities on the other" (McCance et al 1999: 1392).

The theory developed by Leininger (1985), initially a mental health nurse, originated from an anthropological perspective and was labelled 'the theory of cultural care'. Her theory considered the universality and diversity of caring, leading to a culturally sensitive approach in nursing. Watson's theory (1985), again a mental health nurse by background, was based on a form of humanism and has origins in the philosophy of being and knowing, but she also acknowledges the influence of Leininger in her theory development (Cohen 1991). She offered ten carative factors and a focus on transpersonal caring. Her carative factors can be seen to have a strong spiritual element, based in existential phenomenology and humanism. There have been at least forty studies conducted using her theoretical framework, which have had a significant impact on nursing (Smith 2004).

Roach, like Watson, was influenced by the philosophical approach of phenomenology, particularly Heideggerian hermeneutic phenomenology, and also has a clear focus on theology (McCance et al 1999). Watson, though, appears to have been more influenced by the theory of Carl Rogers, the humanist. Roach identified that caring is not unique to nursing but is unique within nursing, which has also been said of midwifery (Lundgren 2004). She conceptualises caring in her 'five Cs': compassion, competence, confidence, conscience and commitment (McCance 1991). Boykin and Schoenhofer's (1993) theory of caring can be seen to reflect some of the views set out by Roach in that they, too, identify caring as a human mode of being. Caring is an essential feature of human beings and it is a shared experience between carer and cared-for. All four of these theories recognise the importance of the relationship between carer and client and highlight an overarching acceptance of humanistic theory in caring (McCance 1999).

Caring from a theological perspective has been labelled 'moderated love' (Campbell 1984, Kendrick and Robinson 2002). In fact there have also been nursing theorists (Freshwater and Stickley 2002, 2004) and midwifery theorists (Hall 2001) who have suggested that the caring relationship is a type of loving relationship. This, though, can create problems for some and so there have been attempts to re-label this caring relationship to remove the sexual implications of this 'moderated love', both sexual stereotyping and romantic love (Campbell 1984, Morrison 1992). Given professional traditions, policies and legislation within which 'moderated love' occurs, it has been suggested that the professional caring relationship is labelled the 'skilled companion' (Campbell 1984).

Kendrick and Robinson (2002) wrote that, instead of reframing loving care, as suggested by Campbell and supported by Morrison, the caring relationship should be accepted as a loving relationship. This type of love would be recognised as *agape,* as accepted within the Christian tradition, and the relational ethic applied. These relational ethical principles of inclusive community, social freedom and equal respect might address the concerns about the sexual views of love.

It is quite interesting that, for some, there is a need to remove any link between sexuality and caring, whilst there is a body of literature that recognises and rejoices in the sexuality of professional midwifery care (Devane 1996, Robertson 2000, Hall 2002, Williams 2004). It may be that midwifery care is different from the types of caring that are seen in other helping relationships.

The caring relationship has been likened to the relationship between mother and child; it has been seen as a mothering relationship. There is a debate within midwifery about whether it is appropriate for midwives to take on a mothering role. Some midwives suggest that it is unhelpful for midwives to 'mother' women becoming mothers (Kirkham 2000) and other caring theorists (Campbell 1984) support this. This is because it is seen as unhelpful to infantilise adults who need help and care. Some midwives, though, suggest the midwife behaving as a 'good mother' towards women becoming mothers, can act as a role model for them and provide support (Hildingsson and Häggström 1999).

Although the relationship between midwife and woman is unique (Lundgren 2004) there are many elements of the care of nurses and midwives that overlap (Way 2000). Indeed, less than a hundred years ago midwifery was seen as a branch of nursing (Leap and Hunter 1993). Therefore, the theories discussed above and the research into nursing care can be helpful to explore when considering the caring undertaken by midwives, as long as there is recognition of the uniqueness of the midwife-woman relationship (Lundgren 2004).

Nursing research informs us that physical nursing activities or care can be seen as an outward symbol of caring and offer a bridge to a woman's or patient's inner world, but to be effective in providing care there is also the need for good interpersonal skills (Morrison 1992). Despite this, a distinction should not be made between 'instrumental' (nursing tasks) and 'expressive' (interpersonal communication) roles within nursing, as both can, and do, have an impact on caring and the achievement of comfort (Benner 1984). This can be seen to relate directly to midwifery's instrumental and expressive care.

For some, the experience of being cared for is an experience of overwhelming vulnerability due, in part, to the health problem that brought them into care, but also to their vulnerability to professional carers. The care environment is not seen for some as a place of comfort but as a place of fear and anxiety (Morrison 1992). To address this, patients develop survival tactics, but also identify their respectful admiration of the nurses. Carers should, therefore, recognise the patient's lifeworld experiences and consider this when providing care. This had been recognised previously and it had been suggested that "caring cannot be controlled or coerced; it can only be understood and facilitated" (Benner 1984: 171). The development of strategies to understand care is important and meanings and commitments should be taken into account, both personal and cultural, for client and carer (Benner 1984).

Caring in midwifery

A significant study was undertaken to explore caring in midwifery by McCourt et al (2000). In part of their main study they interviewed 20 women from a number of minority ethnic groups, who had all given birth in the previous three to six months. The data was analysed using a grounded theory approach. From this group of mothers a number of dimensions and attributes of caring arose. The themes from the analysis were: choice and knowledge (self or expert knowledge), concepts of care and support, communication and information, professional attitudes and relationships with women, continuity of carer, and confidence and trust. From these themes, the six dimensions and attributes of caring, it was identified what these women would have liked in the midwives caring for them. They would have liked the midwives to have an attitude of friendly presence and to respect their knowledge and themselves. The women wanted to be supported psychologically and physically by the midwife, who should offer the kind of help they needed, when they needed it, rather than at the midwives' determination (McCourt et al 2000). The desires of this group of women relate very closely to the four theories of nursing care and the theologian's 'moderated love' or agape.

The women in this study (McCourt et al 2000) felt that care involved reassurance that they would know who was caring for them. The midwives would be able to provide physical and practical care at a high standard and the women would be treated honestly. Along with this, they thought that good communication skills and interest in their pregnancy were elements of caring. Good communication skills in health care professionals have already been identified as necessary (Morrison 1992, Morse et al 1992, Richards 1999) but this study identified the importance for midwifery specifically.

The implications from research studies (Morrison 1992, Morse et al 1992, McCourt et al 2000) and the Government initiatives (NICE 2003, 2006, DoH 2004) are that midwives need to develop relationships with women in which they can demonstrate expertise and good communication skills, along with respect, empathy and interest. Care, including expertise and good communication, is considered to be demonstrated through the midwife-woman relationship.

The midwife-woman relationship

The midwife-woman relationship has been identified as the central element of midwifery care in numerous studies (Fleming 1998b, Fraser1999, Walsh 1999, Pairman 2000, Kirkham et al 2002, McCourt 2005, Hunter 2006). There is also evidence to suggest that the relationship between midwives and women affects the quality of the childbirth experience for women (Anderson 2000, Hunter 2001). Despite the significance of this relationship, it has received little research attention (Hunter 2006). Indeed Kirkham (2000) was surprised when editing her book 'The Midwife-mother Relationship' that a book of its nature was not already available. A browse through the midwifery educational text also demonstrates a lack of focus on this important area of midwifery practice.

In her book, Kirkham and her colleagues explore the nature of the midwife-woman relationship and the confounding factors, such as the driving force within health services where the aim is to achieve the maximum health gain for the minimum use of resources. Developing relationships can be resource heavy and, given that pregnant women are not generally unhealthy, a paradox may occur. In the twentieth century, health provision, including midwifery, was hierarchically organised, with medicine holding the more senior positions with most authority. This could lead to those lower on the hierarchical ladder adhering to, and accepting, the value base of the more dominant groups and suppressing their own values. This is suggested to have occurred within midwifery, leading to the relationships between midwives and mothers becoming in some ways oppressive, with mothers being treated like children (Kirkham 2000).

A caring and supportive relationship between midwives and women can be difficult to achieve and maintain within the current culture in health (Fraser 1999, Levy 1999c, Kirkham 2000, Kirkham et al 2002a, Stapleton et al 2002a). This can lead to stress and tension in midwives (Hunter 2006) and a perception of this work as low status. It would appear that the value of the development of midwife-woman relationships in maternity care is only acknowledged when absent (Kirkham 2000). This can be seen to lead midwives to alienate women from their own experiences in favour of the expert's experience (Wilkins 2000). The lack of opportunity for women-centred care appears to be particularly problematic in large, institutional maternity provision (Hunter 2004). Despite midwifery's traditional knowledge and research knowledge complementing each other, the authoritative knowledge of the organisation appears to prevail (Kirkham 2000).

A review of studies pertaining to the relationship between midwife and woman, although evidence is limited and inconclusive, suggests that, from the woman's perspective, active presence, mutuality and intimacy are pivotal in the development and maintenance of the relationship (Hunter 2006). Evidence regarding the midwives' perspective on this relationship is likewise limited and the studies available suggest that the relationship may be influenced by situational factors and that there may be differences between midwives' reports and women's perceptions (Fleming 1998a, Fleming 1998b, Kirkham et al 2002a, Hunter 2006).

A large study, conducted in New Zealand and the UK, explored the relationships between women and midwives (Fleming 1998a). Two hundred and fifty midwives and two hundred and nineteen women were interviewed and the data analysed, using a grounded theory approach with elements of interpretative phenomenology. The core categories found were attending and presencing, supplementing and complementing, and reflection and reflexivity. Linking the core categories was the social process of reciprocity. There were also found to be discrepancies between the reports of midwives and women (Fleming 1998a). On the whole though, the study does appear to correlate with Hunter's (2006) review, which identified 'attending' as important and the centrality of reciprocity within these midwife-woman relationships.

A qualitative study, using a feminist approach, was also conducted in New Zealand (Fleming 1998b). This study employed individual interviews, videotapes and group interviews with 12 midwives and 20 women. This, like the previous study (Fleming 1998a), was focused on the relationship between midwives and women. Within this study, again, contradictions in the perceptions of the midwives and women on their relationships were found (Fleming 1998b).

Reviewing the literature related to the reciprocal midwife-woman relationship, it is clear there are cultural problems for the midwife trying to undertake this way of working (Kirkham 2000, Wilkins 2000, Hunter 2006). Sadly, even when the midwife does believe she has achieved a reciprocal relationship, it may not be perceived as such by the woman (Fleming 1998a, Fleming 1998b, Kirkham et al 2002a, Hunter 2006). Despite this, both midwives and women appear to need a reciprocal relationship within which midwives offer active presence and intimacy (Fleming 1998a, Hunter 2006).

The different types of midwife-woman relationships have been simplistically labelled reciprocal, unsustainable exchanges, and rejected exchanges (Hunter 2006). Only reciprocal relationships are said not to create emotional work for midwives. The conversational styles within these interactions have been categorised into 'partnership', where midwives are collaborative and participative, 'professional', where midwives provide expert guidance and 'disciplinary', where midwives provide expert surveillance (McCourt 2005). The most common style found to be used by midwives is the professional style, but situational factors did seem to influence how collaborative the interaction was and the midwives seemed unaware of the style they were adopting. It would appear that the disciplinary style is the one most likely to be rejected, given its impact on health promotion (McCourt 2005). The reciprocal relationship and partnership interactional styles intuitively go together. It may be that the effort to achieve this type of relationship leads midwives to adopt the professional style, but this could be unsustainable in the longer term.

Despite the mismatch between midwives' and women's perceptions, it would appear that both recognise the importance of this relationship and the cultural problems associated with it. To develop and maintain therapeutic or trusting relationships it is recognised that the midwife needs to have good communication skills (Morrison 1992, Richard 1999, McCourt et al 2000).

Communication skills

When people, such as midwives and women, come together there is always communication, whether this is directed towards someone or not; it could be the communication of being tired or busy, or perhaps alert and interested (Kirkham 1993). Communication skills are used extensively in midwifery (Kirkham 1993, Pairman 2000), indeed they are one of the three crucial competencies that a new midwife needs (Butler et al 2008). Despite this, there is a lack of clarity about the techniques used (McCourt 2005). Communication is of primary importance to the women but they have had mixed experiences of this in the care they received (Fraser 1999).

A study was undertaken using semi-structured and structured interviews and women's case notes (Fraser 1999). Forty-one women were interviewed during pregnancy, in hospital following birth and in their homes two to three weeks later. These produced data that was analysed, using a software package that facilitates data handling in a method similar to that of grounded theory. Themes were sought, which were grouped into categories and subcategories.

The women all expressed the desire to feel special and for the caregiver to help them relax, to be in control and to advocate for them. Seven of the forty-one women were unhappy with the communication skills of the carer and three were particularly upset with what they saw as "inappropriate attitudes between the professional groups" (Fraser 1999: 103). Although the midwives were seen to be clinically competent, some of the women were critical of the support and information that they were given. Half the women gave up breast feeding, stating that the primary cause was due to inadequate help. Some women also identified that some midwives were task- orientated and that informed choice was just rhetoric.

Communication has been found to be important, regardless of the care setting (Kirkham 1993, Fraser 1999, Walsh 1999). Walsh's study was developed to compare the experiences of women who had previously given birth to their babies supported by conventional care, but this time were cared for within a partnership caseload model of care. Walsh's study (1999) used an ethnographic approach; he interviewed ten women 8-12 weeks after the birth, comparing this scheme with previous experience of conventional care. Within the partnership caseload scheme, the women felt that their relationships with the midwives were personal and intimate and labelled the relationships as friendships. The women felt valued, respected and cared for; some felt empowered and in control. It would appear that, where special schemes like this one are set up to address the recommendations of the Changing Childbirth document (DoH 1993), they are well evaluated, but this may be due to extra resources being made available and more innovative and enthusiastic midwives taking part. Despite the differences in the women's evaluations of care between Fraser's and Walsh's study, communication and the relationship between midwife and woman were said to be important.

The environment in which the relationship is enacted appears to influence communication (Kirkham 1993). When midwives visited women in their homes the atmosphere was more relaxed and conversation more fluid, facilitating the opportunity for the women to ask questions at their own pace (McCourt 2005). A relaxed approach, using general conversation by the women and midwives, can also act as a tool to maintain normality of the childbirth process and to maintain an atmosphere of calm (John and Parsons 2006). Interestingly, this approach can comfort people who are suffering ill-health as well (Williams and Irurita 2004).

For most health care professionals, understanding of their communication skills has developed from psychological theory and research, particularly from the humanist tradition, such as Rogers (1950) and Egan (1977). The humanist approach has already been shown to be influential in the development of caring theories. According to the humanists, there are four core conditions to therapy or therapeutic communication: empathy, genuineness or congruence, warmth, and unconditional positive regard (Stewart 2005: 108). A general adoption of psychological approaches by other health care professionals can, though, be problematic (Morse et al 1992). In particular, the adoption of, and pressure to engage unquestioningly with, the concept of empathy may be a problem. It is questionable whether health care professionals, other than therapists, should accept that there is a need to demonstrate empathy, as this might put too high a burden on them. This might then lead to ill-health or avoidance of care by the professional (Morse et al 1992).

Egan (1977) took the foundational work of Rogers (1950) and developed it to form the role of the 'skilled helper'. He developed both instructors' manuals and student worksheets to facilitate the development of communications skills. Neither Rogers (1950) nor Egan (1977) see these skills to be the exclusive property of psychotherapy; they recognise they can be used by anyone who wishes to help others. There is a wealth of psychological literature pertaining to communication skills, but those from the humanist tradition of psychology are the most commonly taught to health care professionals.

It is clear that communication is a crucial element of showing care. When the care giver communicates effectively, particularly demonstrating positive regard, being honest and warm, the experience of the receiver is enhanced. The areas of listening, touch and information-giving would appear to be particularly significant in midwifery, so these areas will be considered individually.

Listening

> "It is as though he/she listened and such listening as his/hers enfolds us in a silence in which at last we begin to hear what we are meant to be" (Lao-Tse cited Nelson-Jones 1995: 40).

Listening is probably the most important part of communication (Burnard 2002) and there is specific guidance for listening and attending available, particularly in psychological literature (Egan 1977).

Competence in and the ability to develop relationships are both influenced by the listening skills (Hall 2001, Williams and Irurita 2004) as described by Egan (1977). Despite the limited literature available, these appear to be the skills that midwives are using; midwives can be seen to use open-ended questions and focus on the woman to explore and understand the woman's perspective (Lundgren and Dahlberg 2005). Appropriate non-verbal interactions, such as listening, facilitate the feeling of being valued in a patient, which can be seen to play a part in developing personal control and emotional comfort (Kirkham 1993, Hall 2001). The non-verbal abilities that facilitate this feeling of being valued are having eye contact, sitting in close proximity, and displaying gentleness and concern through touch, active listening and smiling (Williams and Irurita 2004).

Communication skills are accepted as being of paramount importance to women, yet some of them have been unhappy with the communication skills of their caregiver in maternity services (Fraser 1999). Women described poor communication skills and included statements such as "she didn't relate to me", and "staff on the ward knocked my confidence". They were also critical of the attitudes of the caregivers and included statements such as "treated me like a naughty child" and "rude and shouted at me". Women identified that good communication involved abilities, such as "able to explain things" and "being a good listener" (Fraser 1999: 102).

Good communication has also been found to improve the experiences of labouring women (Hall 2001, Lundgren and Dahlberg 2005); talking and touching increased comfort and, when a woman is more distressed, purely listening is most helpful (Schuiling and Sampselle 1999). Most of the women in Fraser's study (1999) were impressed with their overall care, but sadly Kirkham et al (2002a) found, when evaluating the implementation of a leaflet, that midwives were focused on tasks, rather than listening to the women.

There is evidence that good communication is not being experienced by all women who access maternity services and listening is probably the most important skill within communication. Therefore, it can be assumed that some midwives are not actively listening to women. There is evidence to suggest that listening is important to facilitate a feeling of being valued (Kirkham 1993, Fraser 1999, Hall 2001, Williams and Irurita 2004) and a feeling of comfort (Schuiling and Sampselle 1999). Gaining respect or being valued is an underlying philosophy of the NSF (DoH 2004) and comfort is stated by the midwives' professional body (NMC 2004) to be the aim of midwives. Listening could therefore be said to be central to midwifery care and will be considered in more detail in chapter four exploring the emotional care given by midwives.

Touch

> "The need to be touched, held, nurtured is with us from the very beginning to the end of our life" (Campbell 1984: 110).

Touch is an important component of the therapeutic relationship along with other non-verbal responses, which could include: postural echo, nodding, smiling and the use of silence (Egan 1977). Touch is an extremely valuable tool when attempting to care for a person, but the carer needs to be sensitive and assess when touch is appropriate (Kirkham 1993, Morse 2000). Within certain cultures, many are uncomfortable with touching those they do not know well, but touch should also depend on the physical and psychological condition of the person, as well as this cultural element.

Alongside the wider societal general culture or hegemony in the US or UK there are a number of other ideologies or belief systems that dictate when touch is and is not appropriate. Some religions give clear rules about who is allowed to touch whom and when, for example Muslim men and women only shake hands with people of the same sex unless they have a close relationship. There are also a number of social sub groups or outcastes referred to as 'untouchable', for example the Dalit in India, with whom touch is avoided.

Touch is seen in health and social care in the UK as something of a minefield with some professionals, fearful of accusation and litigation, now believing that they should avoid it (Pemberton 2010). Professional touch is, though, acknowledged as important within these services. There are no specific laid down rules for touch but professional bodies offer guidance for their registrants. The guidance relates to ensuring that the patient, client, or other person is treated with respect and dignity, facilitating informed decision making and trust (NMC 2008, GSCC 2010).

Touch - suffering

Two types of suffering have been identified and labelled, emotional and enduring suffering, and each appear to need a different approach to touch (Morse 2000). Enduring suffering is where a person shuts off their emotions to cope, whereas emotional suffering is where a person releases their emotions. Enduring suffering is where a person is protecting themselves from suffering and, to provide comfort at this time, carers use strategies to support this to show respect for the person. Strategies usually accessed at this stage are encouragement and praise, whereas, when a person is suffering and emotionally responding to their situation, caregivers physically support the person by hugging, holding and extensively using touch.

Midwives use touch, not only to address observed cues of suffering, but also as a means of developing rapport with women (Kirkham 1993); this calls for extra effort (John and Parsons 2006). They develop rapport, which they believe is an important part of developing a therapeutic relationship, through "basic care, touch, facial encouragement, chit- chat and sharing part of *themselves*" (John and Parsons 2006: 268). Likewise, people who are unwell feel valued and comforted through displays of gentleness and concern by using touch (Williams and Irurita 2004).

Kitzinger (1977) reminds midwives that touch is important in showing care for women. She even identified different types of touch midwives might use, including comfort touch, diagnostic touch and physically supportive touch. It is, though, important to be insightful about when it is appropriate to touch and which type of touch to use (Kitzinger 1977, Morse 2000).

Touch can, therefore, be seen to be an important element of midwives' communication as part of their therapeutic relationships (Kitzinger 1977, Morse 2000, John and Parsons 2006). Whilst there needs to be recognition that touch should be used sensitively, if done so, it may offer considerable comfort to the woman (Kitizinger 1977, Schuiling and Sampselle 1999, Morse 2000, Williams and Irurita 2004, John and Parsons

2006). The experience of touch in relationship to emotional care will be further considered in chapter four.

Another important area in the communication of midwives is information-giving. There is great emphasis from the modern NHS, professional bodies and government guidelines for health care professionals, like midwives, to ensure, as part of their communication with their clients and before commencement of any treatment, that they give accurate information and gain informed consent.

Information giving

Giving information has been widely discussed in midwifery literature, some of which highlights the powerful positions of those who hold information or knowledge (Lomax and Robinson 1996, Levy 1999a, b,c,d,e). Information- giving is highlighted in government guidelines (NICE 2003, 2006, DoH 2004) and it has been identified that information-giving is the main feature of the 'booking visit' (McCourt 2005), which is where women are first registered with maternity services.

Although there is a wealth of literature on communication and information-giving, these terms are singularly unhelpful in understanding what midwives actually do (Robinson and Lomax 1996). To address this concern, conversation analysis has been used to develop a greater understanding (Lomax and Robinson 1996). Videotaped postnatal consultations between midwives and women in both hospital and the women's homes were taken. It was found that, when the data was analysed using a conversation analytical style of data analysis, midwives were not adhering to the woman-centred approach advocated in either hospital or home setting (Lomax and Robinson 1996), unlike findings in previous and subsequent studies (McCourt 2005).

McCourt (2005) conducted a study to explore whether the booking appointment or first appointment for the pregnant woman to meet with the midwife and exchange information, was the same experience for all the women within the same geographical area. This observational study was developed, as there seemed to be an inconsistency between an audit of case notes and the opinions of the women using the service. The audit found no difference between 'caseload' and 'conventional care', whereas the women felt there was a better quality of care within 'caseload care'. Forty appointments were observed and it was found that the interactional style of the midwives was different for 'caseloading' and 'conventional care' (McCourt 2005).

In conventional care in hospital and clinic settings, the interaction styles were led by history- taking, followed by information- giving and then an opportunity to ask questions. It was formalised and structured, whereas the caseload appointments in the women's own homes were quite different, the information- giving and receiving was more fluid and variable (McCourt 2005).

Despite the credibility of McCourt's study (2005), it needs to be accepted with caution, as midwives have been found to take control and set the agenda for the interactions within the midwife-woman communication and information- giving (Lomax and Robinson 1996, Levy 1999b). It was found that midwives dictated the agenda and did not explain it or ask the women for their opinion. In hospital and home visits, the timing of the interactions were decided by the midwives; the women were not given a time for these meetings and they occurred, regardless of what the women were doing. The midwives dictated closure on the interactions with consent assumed, rather than sought. They also did most of the talking. They talked at length while the women attended fully but when the women talked the "midwife did not attend fully to client talk, frequently turning away and writing notes. In fact, given the frequency of this activity by midwives, it would not be unreasonable to suggest that midwives invite clients to speak at length in order that they may accomplish clerical aspects of the visit" (Lomax and Robinson 1996: 254).

Unfortunately, the literature on information-giving shows a lack of consistency, with some suggesting that differences in approach are due to the situation (Walsh 1999, McCourt 2005) and others stating that midwives take control, regardless of the setting (Lomax and Robinson 1996). It is suggested that it can be difficult for women to gain the information they feel they need, due to complex power relationships, which underlie information-giving behaviour (Kirkham 2000, McCourt 2005).

Levy (1999a, b,c,d,e) explored information- giving in her study, and has written a number of papers related to information-giving as a means of developing informed choice. Levy (1999d, e) conducted a study using grounded theory to explore the information-giving practices from the perspective of midwives (1999d) and from the perspective of the women

(1999e). She observed the midwives and women in 12 booking appointments, as in McCourt's (2005) and Lomax and Robinson's (1996) studies, but she also interviewed each of them individually. Levy (1999d, e) found that giving of information is not as simple a process as other studies may indicate (Lomax and Robinson 1996, Walsh 1999, McCourt 2005). She identified powerful forces involved in information- giving, which involved the gate- keeping role taken by midwives and the manipulation of the information- giving agenda by them.

Midwives used a process Levy labelled 'protective steering' to facilitate informed choice (Levy 1999d). This process involved three main activities: orientating, protective gate- keeping and raising awareness. The midwife, in order to undertake this highly complex activity with limited time, 'picked her line' between orientating, gate-keeping and raising awareness. Orientating was where the midwife found out the position of the woman, her expectations, and how these related to the organisation and the midwife through what Levy labelled 'sensitising'. To achieve this within a limited timescale, the midwives accessed techniques, such as 'stereotyping' and 'territory mapping'. The midwife, through setting the agenda for information-giving, elucidating and offering choices, conducted the activity of raising awareness. The other activity undertaken, labelled 'protective gate-keeping' is where the midwives provided information but also guarded and controlled it. This 'protective steering' was undertaken to ensure that safe, realistic and acceptable choices were made for the woman, midwife and organisation.

Information-giving, as has already been established, is a significant part of a midwife's role, so any exploration of what a midwife does, needs to consider this area. Levy's study offers the best available understanding of what may be happening when midwives give information and offers an explanation of why midwives have been found not to give all the available information to women. Her study also offers another insight into the culture in which midwives are offering emotional support or care.

Alongside the process identified as 'protective steering' (Levy 1999d) is a study that offers the experiences of the woman in the same phenomenon. This, process arising from the experiences of women, has been labelled 'maintaining equilibrium' (Levy 1999e). This was explored using grounded theory and the core categories found were actioning, contextualising and regulating information. Each woman maintained equilibrium by dealing with information by actioning, contextualising and regulating it to protect and keep safe herself, the baby and her family, at what was, for her, a time of great transition. In each of the activities of maintaining equilibrium the women used different strategies.

Levy's research (1998a, b,c,d,e) is helpful in offering a deeper understanding of what might be happening in the studies of Lomax and Robinson (1996), Walsh (1999) and McCourt (2005). In their studies (Lomax and Robinson 1996, Walsh 1999, McCourt 2005), women appear to be naive participants or recipients of midwives' advice, which does not appear to be the case in Levy's studies. All of these studies, including Levy's, highlight the powerful position of those holding knowledge or information. Levy offers a view of information- giving and receiving as a complex interaction, with both parties taking active roles with their individual agendas, not one where midwives hold all the power and control.

This allows for a greater understanding of the findings of the evaluation of evidence-based leaflets that were developed to inform choice in midwifery care. The Midwives' Information and Resource Service (MIDIRS) and the NHS Centre for Review and Dissemination, developed 10 research-based information leaflets to help women make decisions on the choices available to them on their journey to motherhood. A number of papers have been published from this evaluation, with O'Cathlain et al's (2002) randomised controlled trial and Stapleton et al's (2002a) qualitative study published in the British Medical Journal. Alongside this, a series of articles were published in the British Journal of Midwifery (Kirkham et al 2002a,b, Stapleton et al 2002b,c). Sadly, the desired improvement of informed choice in midwifery care does not appear to have been achieved and these authors spell out their explanations for this.

The leaflets were not distributed in the way that had been anticipated, due to the culture within maternity services. The hierarchical power structure, which placed obstetricians in the most authoritative positions, led to them defining the norms of practice (Stapleton et al 2002a). The midwives appeared to identify strongly with the medical and organisational power groups to avoid creating problems for themselves and the women they were caring for (Stapleton et al 2002b). They clearly identified the impact of stepping outside of the practice norms set by the medical team and organisation, such as their work being more scrutinised and the women being 'struck off' GP lists (Stapleton et al 2002b). Stapleton et al (2002c) go on to describe how the organisational impediments, such as the midwives' conversational styles, further reduce the opportunity for the change the leaflets might bring. This, together with time pressures and the belief that, in litigious situations, technical interventions would be seen more positively, acted to reduce the impact of the leaflets (Stapleton et al 2002a).

Kirkham et al's (2002a) paper entitled 'Checking not Listening', attempted to explain one element of this major study. They found that midwives were 'checking rather than listening' to women, they were doing obstetric observations rather than listening to the woman's needs, desires and concerns. The article clearly explains this discrepancy and offers the women's perception on why this occurred. The women saw the midwives as overworked and powerless, despite the midwifery rhetoric for woman-centred care. It may also be that midwives were attempting to improve their status by undertaking tasks that were more in keeping with medicine.

It could be suggested that the process of 'protective steering' (Levy 1998d) was being undertaken by the midwives in Stapleton et al's study (2002a,b,c). The midwives could be viewed as guiding the women to gain what they believe is the best they can, within the boundaries of the medical and organisational systems. Elements of 'maintaining equilibrium' (Levy's 1998e) in the women could also be identified in the evaluation of these information-giving leaflets (Kirkham et al 2002a, Stapleton et al 2002a).

The tightrope-walking identified in Levy's studies and Kirkham et al's (2002a) findings add weight to what has been labelled the 'inverse law' in midwifery care (Kirkham 2002b). This 'inverse law' refers to where the midwives stereotyped women into categories. These categories resulted in women of lower social economic classes receiving less information and support, despite recognition that they might need more. Giving information and support took more time and so it was only the women who sought information who were responded to. Interestingly, Kirkham et al (2002b: 509) state "this accommodating style of communication was accentuated if a male professional partner was present". Stereotyping can be seen as negative if it leads to discrimination, but people use it extensively as a shortcut when time is limited (Barker 2007); it may also indicate discrimination and a gender bias (Kirkham et al 2002b).

Whilst information-giving is recognised as an essential part of a midwives' role (DoH 2004, NICE 2004, 2006), there is a lot of discussion about whether accurate information is being given (Kirkham et al 2002a,

Stapleton et al 2002a) and whether this is being undertaken in a woman-centred manner, as stipulated (Lomax and Robinson 1996, Walsh 1999, McCourt 2005). The explanation for this discrepancy may be found in the culture in which midwives are working (Levy 1999d, Kirkham 2000, McCourt 2005, Kirkham 2000) and the needs of women (Levy 1999e). The conclusions drawn from these studies, such as cultural pressures, and that both midwives and women bring agendas to their interactions, can offer insight into other midwifery activities. It is also important to remember that information-giving is one way in which to offer support and provide comfort.

It has been suggested that, despite the importance linked to this part of a midwife's role by government, it may be seen as lower importance to midwives than other activities, such as examination skills (Kirkham 2002a).

Despite the emphasis in ICM competencies (2006), NSF (2004), NICE guidelines (2003, 2006) and other midwifery literature (Fraser 1999, Butler et al 2008) on women-centred, individualised, negotiated care, many foundational midwifery textbooks focus on physical care activities. Johnson and Taylor (2006), along with Way (2000), have no sections or chapters discussing communication or relationships. Other texts, such as Wickham's (2005) and Fraser and Cooper's (2003) midwifery texts, do offer some information on communication and midwife-woman relationships, but it is still limited.

It appears that knowledge of, and skills in, physical processes are considered to be of high importance in the education of midwives. A newly qualified midwife might also be led to believe that this is the main focus of their role, despite the findings of Butler et al (2008).

Summary of Care

The most fundamental concept of midwifery is 'care' and it is regularly used to describe what midwives do (McCourt et al 2000, Stewart 2004, Page and McCandlish 2006). The midwife-woman relationship has been identified as the central element of the 'care' provided by midwives (Fleming 1998b, Fraser1999, Walsh 1999, Kirkham 2000, Pairman 2000, McCourt 2005, Hunter 2006). There is also evidence to suggest that this relationship affects the quality of the childbirth experience for women (Anderson 2000, Hunter 2001), which increases its significance in the midwives' role. A caring and supportive relationship between midwives and women can be difficult to achieve and maintain within the current culture in health (Kirkham 2000) and this can lead to stress and tension in midwives (Hunter 2006).

To develop and maintain the midwife-woman relationship, midwives extensively use their communication skills (Pairman 2000). They are recognised as one of the three crucial competencies that a new midwife needs (Butler et al 2008). Despite this, there is a lack of clarity about the techniques midwives use (McCourt 2005), but there appears to be some indication that they are using the skills described by Egan (1977). Communication is seen as of primary importance to women too, but they have had mixed experiences of this in the care they have received (Fraser 1999).

Some women accessing maternity services (Fraser 1999, Kirkham 2000) have not experienced good communication, including listening, which is an important skill within communication (Burnard 2002). There is evidence to suggest that listening is important to facilitate a feeling of being valued (Kirkham 1993, Fraser 1999, Hall 2001, Williams and Irurita 2004) and a feeling of comfort (Schuiling and Sampselle 1999, Morse 2000, Hall 2001). Likewise, touch can also be seen to be an important element of midwives' communication (Kitzinger 1977, Morse 2000, Hall 2001, John and Parsons 2006). When midwives use their communication skills, particularly touch, sensitively, it offers considerable comfort to the woman (Kitizinger 1997, Schuiling and Sampselle 1999, Morse 2000, Williams and Irurita 2004, John and Parsons 2006).

Information-giving is also recognised as an essential part of a midwife's care (NICE 2003, 2006, DoH 2004). There has been a lot of discussion related to whether accurate information is being given. It has been found that this is not always the case (Kirkham et al 2002a, Stapleton et al 2002a). While some suggest that information is being provided in a woman-centred manner, as stipulated (Walsh 1999, McCourt 2005), there is also evidence that this may not be happening (Lomax and Robinson 1996). The explanation for this discrepancy may again be found in the culture in which midwives are working (Levy 1999e, Kirkham 2000, McCourt 2005) and the needs of women (Levy 1999e).

So far, midwifery care has been considered in a general sense, but the rest of this chapter considers one specific area of this care in more detail and that is emotional care, or emotional support.

Emotions / Emotional

Introduction

The development of theories related to emotions, as with the midwifery evidence base, proliferated in the twentieth century. This was in an attempt to understand, change and manipulate emotions for a variety of reasons.

Emotions:

Most psychological texts guide us to assume emotions are intrinsic to human experience and that they are so closely linked to motivation that they are difficult to differentiate (Sternberg 2000, Gross 2005). Sternberg (2000:403) defines emotion as "a psychological feeling, usually accompanied by a physiological reaction" and motivation as "an impulse, a desire, or a need that leads to an action" (p383) it is easy to see why distinguishing between emotion and motivation is difficult.

Within psychology there are usually considered to be five major accepted approaches to understanding the person (Barker 2007). These are usually identified as biopsychological, psychodynamic, behavioural, cognitive and humanistic approaches, although other environmental approaches, such as evolutionary theory and social anthropological approaches, are also used by psychologists.

Each psychological perspective offers an explanation of emotions. There are the biopsychological theories of James-Lange and Cannon-Bard, the cognitive theories of Schachter and Singer, the psychodynamic theory of Freud, the behavioural theories of Skinner and Bandura, the humanistic theory of Rogers and the evolutionary theory of Darwin. Each varies in the amount of influence that cognition has on the experienced emotion, with some suggesting emotions are mostly instinctual or biological and others that they are learnt responses and determined by history and culture.

The biopsychologists, behavioural, cognitive and evolutionary psychologists have focused on what has been labelled 'basic' or 'primary' emotions.

The basic emotions are organised into four pairs by Plutchik: joy and sadness, disgust and acceptance, anger and fear, anticipation and surprise (Gross 2005). The Psychodynamic theorists, such as Bowlby, "regard love, closeness and attachment as fundamental emotions" (Baker 2007:33).

These theories are attempting to determine what initiates emotional experiences and responses, but when considering emotional care or a caring response to perceived emotions it is important to recognise the understanding of the observer or responder. The interpretation of an emotional expression, such as crying, will be culturally determined, hence influenced by history and the environment. It has long been accepted in Western societies that to show emotions is a sign of weakness and of femininity (Baker 2007). The more educated and developed person does not express emotions (Baker 2007), although even in popular culture Spock (a character from Star Trek who was part Vulcan) never showed emotions and was partly ridiculed for his focus on rational – logical responses.

Midwives may find themselves dealing with the basic emotions or more complex but fundamental emotions in a culture that subjugates those expressing them. Midwives are also emotional beings and emotional behaviours in the women with whom they are working may arouse emotional responses in them. Working with emotions in others and coping with one's own emotions takes effort and can create stress (Sandall 1997) and has been labelled emotional labour or emotion work (Hochschild 1979, Hunter 2006).

The emotion work of midwives is considered in more detail in chapter 6, but this chapter is more concerned with how they provide emotional care to women. Despite this, it is important to recognise that the literature available highlights how the manipulation of emotions can be at great cost to the carer. Midwives can be seen to manage their emotions to facilitate emotional well- being of women; they could be considered to be offering the 'gift' of emotion work (Bolton 2000, Hochschild 2003).

Emotional care

None of the concepts explored in this chapter has had clear definitions but relevant literature has been explored in an attempt to gain some clarity. This chapter has explored some theories of care and discussed care within midwifery services. The main element or vehicle for care provision in midwifery is the midwife-woman relationship. To develop and maintain these, midwives need to use their communication skills, including listening, giving information and touch.

A definition and understanding of emotions is equally problematic, given the different psychological approaches. Despite this, midwives need to work with both basic and complex emotions when caring for a woman's emotional needs. Emotional care may therefore need to be multifaceted. It may include assessment of emotional needs, emotional support, emotional therapeutic labour and emotion work.

Within midwifery there is a limited consensus on what emotional support is and how it should be provided, but women have identified the need for this in a number of areas on their transition to motherhood (Edwards 2000). Women wanted supportive midwifery practices, emotional, spiritual and physical support and supportive qualities in their midwives. Supportive qualities appear to include listening, respect, acceptance and being given clear information. Supportive midwifery practices include providing an environment that focused on a normal birth, reduced fear and increased confidence and trust. These can all be seen as elements of a therapeutic midwife-woman relationship (Kirkham 2000), the core of midwifery care. These have also been recommended throughout the literature in midwifery over the centuries (Rhodes 1995) and are still recommended by midwifery professional bodies (ICM 2006) and government (NSF (DoH) 2004, NICE 2006).

Some have suggested that emotional support is differentiated from other support by its being 'emotionally sustaining', whereas other support is more practically orientated. Emotional support might comprise listening, demonstrating concern and intimacy. It has also been suggested that emotional support might be a more ongoing process rather than a one-off event (Mander 2001). Despite the lack of clarity over the term support and other terms such as social support, emotional support, therapeutic emotional labour or emotional care, all of these terms seem to be aiming for the same goal, which could be labelled comfort.

From reviewing the available literature, emotional support appears to be the actions taken in response to perceived emotional needs. Therapeutic emotional labour can be accepted as the effort a carer puts in to their interactions to help the other person. The term emotional care can, and will for the purposes of this book, be used in a wider context and may include emotional support, the assessment and evaluation of this, emotional labour and emotion work. Emotionally supportive qualities appear to be listening, touch, being respectful, acceptance and being given clear information (Schuiling and Sampselle 1999, Edwards 2000, Morse 2000). These should be undertaken whatever the midwifery task may be, such as clinical examinations (Morse 2000). Supportive midwifery practices as part of emotional care are providing an environment that focuses on the normality of motherhood, including the birth, reduced fear and increased confidence, control and trust (Rhodes 1995, Edwards 2000, Kirkham 2000, NICE 2004, ICM 2006).

CHAPTER FOUR

MIDWIVES' EMOTIONAL CARE OF WOMEN BECOMING MOTHERS

Introduction

An understanding of emotional care was developed using the available literature in chapter 3, but what is going to be considered here, using my study, is the detail of this care from the midwives' perspective.

It has already been acknowledged that there is a need for emotional support, which is part of emotional care and that midwives are in the best position to be able to provide this type of care. Chapter 3 considered what care is and identified how it is provided within the midwife-woman relationship. The chapter concluded with a brief explanation of the current understanding of emotional care.

Using both historical and contemporary literature, it appears that emotional support is a necessary part of the midwives' role. A concise summarisation of their role is to provide care to facilitate women's safe transition through a number of stages to motherhood. To undertake this role fully, midwives need a sound holistic (biology, psychology, sociology, cultural and spiritual) knowledge base, a caring attitude and good communication skills (Butler et al 2008).

The midwives' professional bodies (ICM, RCM), as well as government initiatives (NICE 2003, 2006, NSF 2004), guide the midwife to work in partnership with women. The role laid out for midwives by this guidance is complex and skilful.

Care

As identified in chapter 3, the central concept of midwifery is 'care' and it is regularly used to describe what midwives do (McCourt et al 2000,

Stewart 2004, Page and McCandlish 2006). It is also what the governing body for midwives in the UK, The Nursing Midwifery Council (NMC), states that they do (NMC 2008). Care is a difficult concept to define, but nursing and theological theories of care suggest it is part of human nature; it is a humanist response (McCance et al 1999) and can be considered a form of love (Campbell 1984, Kendrick and Robinson 2002, Freshwater and Stickley 2002, 2004). Central to the provision of midwifery care is the midwife-woman relationship (Fleming 1998b, Fraser 1999, Walsh 1999, Pairman 2000, McCourt 2005, Hunter 2006). This relationship not only provides the basis for care-giving; it also affects the quality of the childbirth experience for women (Anderson 2000, Hunter 2001). The centrality of the midwife-woman relationship can clearly be seen in the descriptions that can be found in my study.

Midwife-woman relationship

All the midwives in my study described their relationships with the women they were caring for, when explaining their emotional support. The relationships initially did not run smoothly for them and there was little evidence, in the beginning, of reciprocity to facilitate a mutually gratifying care experience (Fleming 1998a, Hunter 2006). This can be seen by some of the struggles the midwives encountered and which are discussed in chapter 5.

Despite this, the midwives did eventually gain a more reciprocal relationship but it took, as Hunter (2006) would predict, some emotion work. All of the midwives in my study can be seen to be putting effort into their relationships, particularly their communications. Betty needed to put effort into communicating and made extensive use of non-verbal communication behaviours, whereas Carol, Fiona and Emily struggled with understanding the women for whom they were caring. Diane struggled with finding the right way of helping, and communication again became difficult. Gina, in a very stressful but exciting situation, rapidly developed a therapeutic relationship and Hetty took on what could be considered a more maternal role.

All of these midwives' relationships could be considered to be 'unsustainable exchanges', as identified by Hunter (2006) except, perhaps, for Emily, whose relationship may fall into the category of 'rejected exchange' (Hunter 2006). Using McCourt's (2005) styles of conversation, it can be seen that the midwives were using different approaches. Despite all the midwives suggesting they wanted to work in a partnership manner (Partnership: participative or collaborative) with the women, this is not apparent in their interactions. Certainly Carol, Emily and Gina appear to be trying to use this approach, although still showing signs of the professional approach. Betty and Hetty could be seen to be using a professional style (professional: expert guidance) and Diane may even be perceived to be disciplinary from the woman's point of view (disciplinary: expert surveillance). Despite the differing styles at the beginning of the relationships, all the midwives, except perhaps Hetty, who appeared to continue to have a motherly or professional relationship with the woman, appeared to indicate that the relationships became more reciprocal and partnership-like towards the end of their interactions. The changes in the relationships appear to be due to the emotion work invested by the midwives.

It has been recognised that midwives are providing care within competing ideologies, which is explored in more detail in chapter 5, and this can make developing and maintaining the midwife-woman relationship difficult to achieve within the current culture in health (Kirkham 2000). It can also lead to stress and tension in midwives (Hunter 2006). Despite this, it can be seen that the midwives in my study, when they perceived the need for emotional support, used time and effort to develop an intimate relationship with the women they were caring for.

Physical proximity

Close physical proximity can be a means by which to create a feeling of comfort, but this proximity could be influenced by cultural expectations (Williams and Irurita 2004). It is generally assumed that the British public need a greater personal space than other Europeans, but it is necessary at times, within midwifery and nursing, for these cultural expectations to be put on one side. This could be considered to create a paradox in that close proximity facilitates comfort, but invading a person's personal space could lead to embarrassment and discomfort.

Physical proximity was recognised as a necessary part of most midwives' role but it may be found that this is an area for which they need to offer emotional support, as the midwives in this study identified how intimate this proximity was. As part of this support, the inner knowing and close midwife - woman relationship may help to overcome the embarrassment felt by midwives or women, due to this proximity.

The midwives had close physical contact with what is generally considered the most private parts of a woman's body, sight and touching of which is usually kept for her sexual partner. The vaginal examination, which is part of their role, has been identified as an activity that can create anxiety for both midwife and woman and can be distressing, uncomfortable and embarrassing for the woman. The transition of the vagina from an area of sexual pleasure, which is explored in private, to a functional area that is open to inspection from strangers, can be particularly difficult for all involved. Partners can be seen to turn away so as not to watch vaginal examinations and midwives can be seen to use coping strategies, such as infantilising the women (Devane 1996).

The vaginal examination can also be seen as one of the themes of suffering when considering comfort in the violated body (Morse et al 1994). To create comfort in this situation, people tend to distance themselves from what is happening, and when they cannot achieve this, caregivers can help create comfort through presence and connection using their voices, hands and eye contact. We will see later in this chapter that these are techniques used by the midwives in my study.

The close physical proximity experienced by the midwives in my study were clearly described by Gina, who said, *"she had got out of the bath and sat on the toilet she had nothing on when we arrived"* and she went on to explain that she needed to exam the woman's vaginal area *"so I prepared her for this internal examination"*. Gina was concerned about whether this would be uncomfortable for the woman and attempted to maintain the woman's privacy and dignity.

It is not just pregnancy and birth that have sexual elements; the breasts are for most couples a part of sexual interactions and this can lead to relationship problems if a woman is breast-feeding (Devane 1996, Hall 2002). Diane talked of touching the woman's breasts, she said, *"She was quite sore and so I thought we could try with a nipple shield and we tried to get the baby on the breast with the shield"*. The physical proximity did not seem to concern Diane or the woman, whereas the amount of physical assistance needed and given did.

These physical interactions were not undertaken to provide emotional support, but can be seen to be part of providing holistic care, including emotional care. The midwives did not describe how this physical proximity enhanced the emotional support they gave; they appeared to suggest that emotional support was needed by the women, due to the need for physical contact. Gina, in particular, described her behaviours to emotionally care for the woman whilst undertaking these activities, which included eye contact, hands, voice and her presence as indicated above.

Williams and Irurita (2004) acknowledged close physical proximity as a means by which to create a feeling of comfort, but they also pointed out that this proximity could be influenced by cultural expectations. Hunter (2006) indicates the sexual nature of childbirth as another element of midwifery care that may provoke embarrassment and discomfort. She believed midwives should acknowledge this sexual component of childbirth and recognise that it may cause emotion work for them as they attempt to provide appropriate care. Also, sexual behaviour, such as kissing, cuddling, nipple and clitoral stimulation can start and progress labour through hormonal release (Robertson 2000). This did not, though, appear to be an area of concern for the midwives in my study and the midwives appeared quite comfortable with discussing the intimate nature of their contact with the women.

Intimate relationship – use of self

The intimate nature of the relationship between midwife and woman has been recognised by a number of writers (Walsh 1999, Pairman 2000, Hunter 2001, Kirkham et al 2002, McCourt and Stevens 2009). This relationship, as has already been recognised, provides the conduit through which midwives provide their care, including emotional care. It has also been acknowledged in a number of studies that, within this intimate relationship, midwives use something of themselves, self-disclosure (Kirkham 2002, Hunter 2006, John and Parsons 2006) or intuition (Fleming 1998, Hildingsson and Häggström 1999, Callister and Freeborn 2007, Ólafsdóttir 2009, Bone 2009). Hunter (2001) acknowledged the intimate nature of the midwife-woman relationship and explained that this was part of the emotion work of midwives.

Despite the midwives in my study sharing personal information about themselves, they, as was found in a previous study (Kirkham et al 2002b), chose to omit discussing personal birth experiences. This may be due to pressure for midwives to give the 'good answer' expected by the organisation on this particular topic (Kirkham et al 2002b). This could suggest, again, that midwives' practice, including those in this study, is being influenced by the 'being professional / with institution' ideology.

The midwives, though, did not identify this as a reason for not sharing this part of themselves; they suggested it was due to all births being different.

In Hunter's study (2006), self-disclosure became an important element of the midwife-woman relationship and where this was balanced – a reciprocal relationship – the midwives incurred less emotional toll and more job satisfaction. Although Fleming (1998a) does not discuss disclosure, she does identify that interdependence occurs and that the social process of reciprocity is key to this therapeutic relationship. She also identifies midwives as seeking to use intuition, or a sixth sense, to guide their care.

Intuition

Hildingsson and Häggström (1999: 85) described the midwives in their study using intuition, or some other interpretative tool, as "they heard something between the words the woman said…". When they discussed this intuition it was related to how the needs of the women were identified. The use of intuition has been found in other studies (Callister and Freeborn 2007, Ólafsdóttir 2009) and was found in my study as well. Intuition appears to guide the midwives' care and gives them a sense of what is needed and how things will be.

Three ways of intuitive-knowing have been identified:; intuition based on practice experience, intuition based on spiritual awareness and intuition based on connectiveness with women, but these are recognised as overlapping and interrelated (Ólafsdóttir 2009). Inner knowing, based on practice experience, is where the practitioner internalises the knowledge derived from clinical experience and then uses this at a subconscious level. This appears to be what Gina was describing when she talked of using her intuition. She said, *"I think there comes an intuition about when things are going right or when things are going wrong*". She indicated that this intuition came from her numerous experiences and it guided her behaviour. Although she could not clearly identify which experiences led to her understanding of individual situations, *"I can't pinpoint what instinctively makes me feel"*. Hetty said, *"I always trust what my gut is saying that's what it is about and you know I suppose it is part of a spacious relationship"*. It would appear that Hetty is describing intuition, based more on connectiveness with women. It is quite interesting that Hetty had the least partnership-like relationship but appears to be more connected to the woman. It may be, given Hetty's more maternal interactions with the woman, that a motherly relationship develops these apparently closer bonds.

None of the midwives in my study appeared to describe intuition based on spiritual awareness, but this may be due to some of the issues raised by the midwives in Ólafsdóttir's study (2009), particularly that people would think they were crazy. Despite this, the midwives did describe having close relationships with the women they were offering emotional support to, and it may be that, given the level of intimacy, they may have shared more connectiveness and spiritual awareness than has been explicitly identified in their descriptions.

Midwifery literature acknowledges the use of self, whether through self-disclosure or intuition, to develop the midwife-woman relationship and to show care. It is acknowledged that this use of self is undervalued and gains little or no status (Bolton 2000, Kirkham 2000, John and Parsons 2006). The midwives in my study did not appear to seek value and status in offering this type of care, as was seen in the midwives in Cattrell et al's study (2005). The midwives appeared to be seeking permission from some undisclosed authority and the time in which to offer it. Despite this, as it is recognised that emotional support or care is part of a midwife's role, if this type of care was given more status and valued by women (Bolton 2000, John and Parsons 2006) and midwifery services (Kirkham 2000), it might reduce the emotion work of midwives.

The literature shows that, to develop and maintain the midwife-woman relationship, through which they offer emotional care, midwives need to extensively use their communication skills (Pairman 2000). Despite this, there has been a lack of clarity about the techniques midwives use (McCourt 2005). The midwives in my study can be seen to extensively use their communication skills and described in detail the skills they were using to develop and maintain their midwife-woman relationships.

Communication skills – non-verbal

Sadly, it has been found that some women do not experience good communication skills in the midwives caring for them (Fraser 1999, Kirkham 2000), but the midwives in my study described using the skills proposed by theorists and trainers, such as Rogers (1951) and Egan (1977), most of the time.

Non-verbal interactions, such as listening, can facilitate the feeling of being valued, which can be seen to play a part in developing personal control and emotional comfort (Kirkham 1993, Hall 2001). The non-verbal abilities that facilitate this feeling of being valued are: having eye contact, sitting in close proximity and displaying gentleness and concern through touch, active listening and smiling (Williams and Irurita 2004).

Listening

Listening is probably the most important communication skill (Burnard 2002) and the midwives recognised and described undertaking this behaviour. Listening is important to facilitate a feeling of being valued (Fraser 1999, Williams and Irurita 2004) and a feeling of comfort (Schuiling and Sampselle 1999, Morse 2000). Egan (1977) describes active listening as a technique to therapeutically engage with others in a helping relationship, such as the midwife-woman relationship. Active listening involves attending to what the other person is communicating and Egan proposed micro activities to promote this. These micro activities have been labelled using the acronym 'SOLER'. S is to sit squarely, upright and not slouching, to encourage the perception of interest and attention. O stands for open posture, a closed posture of crossed arms or legs can be viewed as a physical barrier to conversation. L means to lean slightly forward and, as long as this does not invade the speaker's personal space, it can demonstrate the desire to hear. E is for eye contact; this needs to be consistent but not to the extent of staring. R is to encourage the listener to appear relaxed; if the listener appears tense this may be interpreted as anxiety and the speaker may respond to this by ending the communication (Rungapadiachy 1999). Facial expression and head movements are also important to demonstrate attention (Hadland 2004).

The midwives in my study all used unobtrusive interactions, such as listening. Carol clearly articulated this perceived need for being heard or listened to in her statement, *"She needed a lot of listening…lots of support"*. Carol also pointed out that listening to the women's stories was not a chore because she enjoyed hearing what the woman had to say. Along with the other midwives Hetty acknowledged the importance of listening. She said she felt that she created her caring relationship by listening. Hetty said she needed to listen to the woman, as it was *"her body, baby and world"*, so it was important that she listened to the woman's perceptions. Some of this sentiment appeared to be shared by Diane, who said, *"She didn't have to listen to everything I was telling her, it was her baby and she knew it in a way that I never do"*. For Hetty, this listening also allowed her to gain a sense of what was happening which, she said was important when offering care.

However, Carol did say that during this time of listening she wrote notes, some of which were necessary for her records but others to give the woman time to talk. As well as taking notes during times of 'listening', the midwives also described listening whilst undertaking other activities, such as physical examinations.

Most of the midwives identified using the routine physical examinations and assessments, in their attempts to recognise and support the woman with her emotions. They felt this relaxed the woman and then the woman felt more comfortable and started to disclose her worries. They went on to say the women identified issues that concerned them during routine physical examination when they were more relaxed. As stated by Emily, *"Very often during the examination they will come out with things"*.

This approach is probably not what Egan would identify as active listening and, although the midwives believed note-taking and physical examinations facilitated a feeling of comfort, or a 'relaxed attitude', this is not upheld by other midwifery studies (Lomax and Robinson 1996). Savage (2004) also suggests that it may not be a sense of relaxation that facilitates the women disclosing problems when being physically examined, but a feeling of vulnerability. Physical examination and the removal of clothes may be a removal of a defence or barrier to disclosure; when the clothes are removed and the bodies seen, so are the emotions exposed.

Despite this, evidence suggests it is not what is done but the way in which it is done that is important in emotional care. Clinical activities, such as physical examination and the observation of vital signs, can all offer a sense of comfort (Morse et al 1994). Morse et al (1994) stress it is not the activity of care that is important, it is the way in which it is undertaken. If it is undertaken 'for' and 'with' the person instead of 'to' them, it restores their integrity and assists in moving them towards recovery. This would also appear to be the aim of women-centred care in midwifery. The midwives appeared to be aiming to work 'for' and 'with' the women they were caring for. An example is where Diane was working 'for' and 'with' the woman to overcome some of her struggles. She said,

> "We um talked it through to deal with that and um we talked through coping with the baby being awake at night and tips for that, just sitting and talking about getting enough sleep and making sure she was getting enough sleep during the day time".

The midwives usually described undertaking physical examinations and clinical observations in a caring manner, which may be considered emotionally supportive (Bone 2009). This can be seen in Gina's descriptions,

> "I was giving her eye contact, looking at her face, I was ignoring the rest of the people in the room" and "I took her hand to offer her some physical attention, I said to her 'do what you want to do'".

Touch

Touch, along with listening, is recognised as an important non-verbal communication skill (Kitizinger 1977, Morse 2000, John and Parsons 2006). When midwives use their communication skills, particularly touch, sensitively, it offers considerable comfort to women (Kitizinger 1977, Schuiling and Sampselle 1999, Morse 2000, Williams and Irurita 2004, John and Parsons 2006). The midwives in my study described many occasions where they used touch in a sensitive manner to support the women they were caring for. Betty described holding the woman's hand and hugging her to develop their relationship and improve the woman's self- esteem and Gina described holding the woman's hand to support her. Indeed, many writers suggest that, if touch is used sensitively, it can facilitate comfort and understanding (Kitzinger 1977, Morrison 1992, Morse 2000, Williams and Irurita 2004, John and Parsons 2006).

Therapeutic touch has been said to enhance a feeling of comfort, peace and calm (Hayes and Cox 1999). Newell et al (1997: 253) state that touch is a "key primal instinct" and an important element of mother-baby interactions. It could be suggested that Betty and Gina were responding to perceived emotional needs, through an instinctual response and the response that reassures babies also reassures and induces peace and calm within adults too. Betty said, *"At the end of that particular visit, as I did for all the others, I gave her a cuddle which drew us close together and it made her feel, I think, that she wasn't being ostracised"*. Betty explained that, as described by John and Parsons (2006), she developed a rapport with the women through her use of touch.

The midwives could be seen to be trying to achieve comfort in the women to whom they offer emotionally supportive care, which they are doing through their use of their non-verbal skills, especially listening and touch (Schuiling and Sampselle 1999, Morse 2000, Williams and Irurita 2004).

Communication skills – verbal

Communication, particularly verbal communication and specifically information- giving, is recognised as an essential part of a midwife's role (NICE 2003, 2006, DoH 2004) and the midwives in my study described at length their information- giving.

There has been a lot of comment in midwifery literature related to whether informed decision- making is being fully supported by midwives. It has been found that, despite there being a great deal of information to support decision- making in becoming a mother, this has not always been given accurately to women (Kirkham et al 2002a, Stapleton et al 2002a). While some suggest that information is being provided in a woman-centred manner, as stipulated (Walsh 1999, McCourt 2005), there is also evidence that this may not be happening (Lomax and Robinson 1996). The explanation for this discrepancy may again be found in the culture in which midwives are working (Levy 1999d, Kirkham 2000, McCourt 2005) and the needs of women (Levy 1999e).

Information giving

Facilitating choice and control are key issues in midwifery care, in line with government directives (particularly Changing childbirth - DoH 1993), and using information-giving to support and empower women has been identified in research studies (Levy 1999a, 1999b, 1999c, McCourt 2005). This appears to be influential in the care given by the midwives in my study. Although it is important to be aware, as Lomax and Robinson (1996) pointed out, that information- giving is quite an ambiguous term.

These midwives can be seen to be caught in the dilemmas found in a number of studies of when, what and how to give information. Some give the information they think is needed, when they think it is needed, as with the midwives in Levy's study; this was labelled 'protective steering' (Levy 1999d). This was discussed in more detail in chapter 3.

All the midwives described their information-giving activities. Despite apparent similarities, there appear to be subtle differences in their approaches. This can particularly be seen in Hetty and Gina's information-giving. Hetty did not appear to be demonstrating a belief in the woman's ability, which is considered important to develop a woman's autonomy (Hildingsson and Häggström 1999). Despite this, Hetty said she was guiding the woman to make good choices in what may be considered to be a similar approach to the midwives in Hildingsson and Häggström's study (1999) where the midwives took on the role of 'good mother'. She may also be considered to be enacting 'protective steering' or 'picking the line' (Levy 1999d), where midwives attempted to meet the wishes of women steering them through dilemmas, by managing their information-giving.

Gina's motivation for information-giving appears to be twofold: she was giving information to gain informed consent, as well as offering choices to reduce the risk of emotional distress later. It could be suggested that Gina's lack of 'protective steering' (Levy 1999d) for the woman created extra stress and reduced her ability to make decisions, given Gina's acknowledgment that the woman was only able to respond at an instinctual level at her stage of labour. Gina said,

> "She was too far advanced to be able to make many decisions but I felt I was making her feel that she was in control and trying to accommodate her wishes" and "in retrospect it would have been very difficult (for her) to have a rational decision, a full conscious thinking decision".

Gina identified that *"they can get extremely distressed post-natally because it wasn't the birth they had planned and um I was maybe trying to forestall this as well. I had experienced that before with this kind of scenario"*.

There seems to have been limited 'protective steering' occurring in Gina's information-giving, but there were clear indications of her applying the 'changing childbirth' guidance. She was promoting control and choice by offering the woman more information than she could, in hindsight, process.

'Protective steering' can, though, be easily seen in Emily's statement,

> "Well I invited her to classes that we run in the area; specifically to the classes we run in that area. Lots of the women get choices, so they can go to the hospital or go to local classes or NCT but I felt for her it would

better to come to the local ones, where she could meet the other women who were pregnant and living in the same area, people living near her and so she agreed to come to those".

This behaviour could also be seen in Betty's descriptions, but her reason for 'protective steering' could be seen to be different. Betty recognised that the woman she was caring for wished to breast-feed and, despite Betty's belief that this would not be a problem, she apparently chose not to inform the woman of this as the paediatrician had informed the woman that she should not breast feed. There appeared to be an implied expectation that Betty should not work against the organisational hierarchy. This is explored more in the next chapter, when considering ideologies and 'toeing the organisational line'. Betty said,

"The lady also wanted to breast feed and although I, as a midwife, could say that research shows that it possibly, probably could have been ok……. She had been strongly advised by paediatricians that she was absolutely not to and so from that point of view she needed quite a bit of support in that".

This also correlates with Stapleton et al's papers (2002b,c); they identified that midwives were impeded from offering certain information due to organisational impediments (2002c) and that they fell in line with medical and organisational power-holders (2002b). It was suggested that midwives did this to protect the women (protective steering by Levy 1998d) and to protect themselves (Stapleton et al 2002b).

Despite the identified 'protective steering', all the midwives described information-giving when they understood the focus was on emotional support. This could lead to the understanding that the midwives saw information-giving as playing a significant role in emotional support. It is generally assumed that, to have information allows for informed choices and a feeling of control, which is advocated by both midwifery literature (Kirkham et al 2002a) and government policy (DoH 1993). This, also, can be seen as part of the belief system of the midwives and appears to have some of its foundations in the Changing Childbirth document (DoH 1993).

Choice, control and continuity appear to be a mantra adopted by the midwives. As part of this, information-giving is said to be pivotal. Whether this is what has led the midwives in my study to discuss information-giving at length or not, it can be seen to play a part in the literature associated with emotional support and comfort (Morse et al 2000, McCourt et al 2000, Williams and Irurita 2004).

McCourt (2005) identified in her study that conversation and information-giving in the home setting was more flexible, fluid and variable. All the midwives in my study chose to offer emotional support in the woman's own home and if, as McCourt suggests, it is more flexible and fluid in this setting, that could account for the wide range of information-giving that was discussed. The differences may also be due to the differing reasons for offering emotional support.

Talking - chatting

Bone (2009) found that it was difficult to distinguish between emotional support and just chatting. Chatting has been identified as a technique for offering emotional support in midwifery (John and Parsons 2006), so there may not be any need to differentiate between them. Chatting, by Cheepen in 1988, and chit-chat, by Hudson in 1980, were labelled as phatic communion (Coupland et al 1992). Phatic communion or communication was a concept developed by Malinowski in the 1920s. He stated that it is the language used in free, aimless social intercourse facilitating sociability and social ties or unions (Coupland et al 1992).

Since its first inception phatic communication has been explored by both sociolinguists and psycholinguists with many viewing it as negative. The underlying hegemony of capitalism and paternalism within western societies puts a higher value on the types of communication that are focused, goal orientated and factually accurate. Conversely phatic communication has been seen as more similar to 'gossip' which along with its lack of focus on veracity is also considered to be a female trait.

It can be recognised, though, from the writings of social psychologists including Goffman (1959, 1970) that phatic communication can play an important role in establishing social 'frames' for individual 'roles'. Laver conducted a number of studies examining phatic communication in the 1970s and '80s and he also offers a positive evaluation of this style of language. He states that it offers a starting point for social interactions and the opportunity to develop relationships (Laver 1975).

The findings of Laver can clearly be seen in the midwives in my study; they were sitting and talking or chatting at the beginning of their meeting which they said by the end of their interactions had come 'full circle' back to chatting at the end. Using the terminology of the sociolinguists, the offering of emotional support started and ended with phatic communication.

Chatting or phatic communication appeared to be different from listening and information-giving, despite both being part of this activity. Emily explained that sitting and talking about general things helped to build the relationship. She said,

> "Just sitting there and having a cup of tea with her, not necessarily chatting about the pregnancy, chatting about the house and work they are doing on it and which is nothing to do with midwifery".

This chatting facilitated a feeling of closeness and normality, encouraging a relaxed atmosphere.

Despite this relaxed approach Emily was still conscious of her behaviour and thought about how she was communicating at a verbal and non-verbal level. She explained how she ensured she did not disclose certain things about herself, particularly her own pregnancies, was mindful of the importance of where she sat and what she was wearing. Fiona and Betty, too, described this way of showing care; they said they simply sat down and had a cup of tea and talked about general things.

Fiona went on to say she did this to develop a comfortable atmosphere, moving slowly onto questions and examinations and when the visit ended they returned to general conversation; it had come "full circle".

> "Basically what I did was something quite simple really, was to go and sit down with a cup of tea and chat about the dogs and things, things that were familiar to her and with which she felt comfortable" .

As can be seen in the above statements, the midwives in my study were giving emotionally supportive care to women in their own homes. This was clearly a decision made by the midwives in their support of women. This is supported by other literature which will be explored later in this chapter. Providing emotionally supportive care in the women's own home, along with the need to offer continuity, choice and control, appears to be part of the midwives' ideological stance. This can be seen to be related to 'with woman' care, or putting the woman at the centre of care, but is not an explicit part of this ideology.

Home-visiting

None of the midwives described giving emotional support anywhere except the home situation and said that, when they recognised the women needed emotional support, they organised a home visit. They clearly believed that home-visiting was a necessary part of offering emotional support, and they gave firm explanations for this belief.

The reasons offered for home-visiting were that it facilitated relationship development; it allowed women to be more comfortable and moved the perceived power from the midwife, giving control to the woman. For example Emily said,

> "It was valuable because we spent an hour together and so I think it built a bit of a relationship for us, whereas if she had come to see me in the surgery we might have had 15 minutes" and "I think people in their own homes tend to feel more relaxed because they are more in control".

It is acknowledged by a number of writers that there is power associated with midwifery knowledge and values, which are recognised by women and midwives (Fleming 1998a). However, Kirkham et al (2002) found that women perceived that midwives had very little control and the power was with the doctors. This could support the Professional and Disciplinary interactive styles (McCourt 2005) discussed earlier in this chapter. The midwives in my study suggested that home-visiting addressed this power imbalance and allowed the women to receive the emotional support they needed, but this was not always achievable due to workload pressure. It has been said that community-based maternity provision equates with caring and hospital-based maternity services equates with curing (McCourt and Percival 2000).

All of the emotional support described by the midwives in my study was conducted in the woman's own home. Information-giving in the home environment was found to be flexible and adapted to the woman, and proceeded as a conversation where the woman was given time to seek the information she needed (McCourt 2005). This also appears to be the case for my study; the midwives were flexible in their approach to information-giving and this was adapted to the women's needs, despite the recognition that they may also be using 'protective steering'.

Home-visiting was thought to improve health and developmental outcomes of the baby, but this was not supported by Doggett, Burrett and Osborn

(2007), in their Cochrane Review of home-visiting of pregnant women who had drug and alcohol-abuse issues. They suggested that there was insufficient data to suggest that home-visiting was beneficial for the mothers' and babies' health. Although Doggett et al (2007) identified a lack of evidence to support home-visiting, facilitating the well-being of women and their babies, there are studies, which did not fulfil the criteria of the Cochrane Review, (Kitzman et al 2000, 1998, Olds et al 2002, 2004), that support the view of the midwives in my study.

To offer home-visiting in the antenatal period is not general practice in the UK (Walsh 1999). However, in the few published studies where this does occur, it is well evaluated by the women (Walsh 1999, McCourt 2005). Fleming (1998b), in her study in New Zealand, also found that women appreciated having antenatal appointments at home.

Walsh (1999) pointed out that women in his study appreciated the home visits in the antenatal period, as they gave the partners and other children the opportunity to get involved. Some of the midwives also recognised the importance of involving partners, some of whom needed support, and others supported the midwife in offering emotional support.

The midwives in my study valued home-visiting to give emotional support to women becoming mothers. Despite this, midwives like Fiona identified that she did not have the time to conduct the home visits she would like, and the NICE guidelines for antenatal care (NICE 2003) appear to make little room for this activity.

> "Not antenatally, because my timetable just does not permit it because I can see 8, 10 women in clinic in a morning whereas if I visit 8, 10 women at home, the time taken travelling between the two I would just never be able to cope with the number of hours that would involve".

This belief by the midwives in my study, when trying to comply with NICE guidelines, could create extra struggles in their providing emotionally supportive care. This is especially so when it is recognised that the guidelines from NICE stipulate who is and is not at higher risk and therefore in need of extra appointments. This is particularly significant, as the midwives identified that it was not always those women who fit at-risk stereotypes who need extra support. They identified that it was difficult to assess who would need extra care and who would not.

One midwife – one woman (continuity of care)

The midwives and at least one of the women (as perceived by her midwife) in my study believed that continuity of care should consist of one midwife caring for a woman throughout pregnancy and into the early days after the birth. This is in contrast to Fleming (1998a) who suggests that there does not need to be a continuous relationship throughout pregnancy and birth, as strong relationships can develop very quickly. She states it is more important to gain a trusting relationship through an interdependent or reciprocal relationship. In support of Fleming's (1998a) findings it has been found that, when people are in states of heightened anxiety, they find the people they come into contact with more attractive. One of the most powerful factors influencing affiliation is anxiety (Gross 2001).

Green et al (2000), in their review of continuity of care, suggest that there has been no firm definition of what constitutes continuity. They suggest continuity of care means care that is not fragmented, which is what they identify that women do not want. Continuity of care, though, has been seen to mean continuity of carer (Green et al 2000), with some recognising this to mean midwifery care being given by one midwife, as indicated by the midwives in my study. The continuity of care message was developed from women consistently saying they "did not like fragmentation, inconsistency, long waiting times and being treated like a number. They wanted to be treated with respect and dignity" (Green et al 2000: 186).

Continuity of carer was seen to be a way of overcoming fragmentation of care and a method for developing a relationship between carer and woman, to allow mutual respect to develop. Continuity of carer may seem to be focusing on one element of what women were saying, when another may be more important to them. Many studies support Green et al's (2000) assertion that what is important to women is to be treated with respect and dignity and that they want to feel special (Fraser 1999, Walsh 1999, McCourt et al 2000).

Continuity of care was an element of care recommended in the Changing Childbirth report (DoH 1993). Since this time, it would appear that continuity of care has become part of the underlying philosophy of midwifery practice (Pairman 2000) and one that appears to be accepted into the belief system of the midwives in my study. There does not appear to be any evidence that what the midwives hold as important – continuity of care – is not so. There is, though, evidence to suggest that it puts increasing pressure on an already pressured midwifery service (Sandell 1997, Green et al 2000).

Time

Giving women time was identified, by the midwives in my study, to be an important part of providing emotional support to women on their journey to motherhood. This is supported by other related literature, such as Morse and Bolton's studies with nurses. Morse, in her studies of providing comfort, identifies time as one of the three most important elements (Morse 2000) and Bolton (2000) also recognises the importance of time when giving 'the gift' of emotion work. Likewise, John and Parson (2006) and Hildingsson and Häggström (1999) identify the need for the resource of time in midwives providing support. Hildingsson and Häggström (1999) also highlight that the midwives in their study not only used their professional time to offer support, but also sometimes used their personal time.

Finding time within their regular working hours and abiding by professional expectations was a struggle for the midwives in my study, as with those in Hildingsson and Häggström's (1999) study. Their appointments appeared to be conducted within fixed time constraints, as was stated by Emily. She said,

> "If she had come to see me in the surgery, we might have had 15 minutes umm you know there wouldn't have been enough time really".

The midwives indicated that providing emotional care took more time than would be expected at a regular appointment, but giving time was an important element of showing this type of care. Fiona, when she was aware that the woman she was caring for needed this extra support, offered her time before approaching questions that she needed to ask about the pregnancy. Fiona explained that the care she gave this woman did not impinge on her personal time, but that there are occasions where she would allow her support to use personal time. Betty and Hetty both talked of working outside their normal hours, giving extra time to the women they were caring for. Betty said, *"That's the most important, we have never ever cut back on the time allowed her"*. She believed that giving time and individualised care was essential. Betty felt, though, that due to the autonomy she has within her role, she was able to achieve giving the woman the time she needed.

Hetty, too, felt giving time was important and said that she did not put a time limit on her visits, which she thought was important but this meant she was sometimes late for her next appointment. Carol, along with Betty, identified the autonomy within her role; she explained how she had the ability to control the time available to her to support the women she was caring for. Carol went on to explain that she could extend the visiting period from 10 days up to 28 days for women *"Who are not quite sure of themselves, not quite comfortable with themselves"*.

Gina and Betty explained how they also needed to spend time talking to the husband to reassure him, when they could have been focused on attending the woman. They felt that, by doing this, it would enhance their ability to give the woman the emotional care she needed.

Time was limited and the midwives explained how offering emotional support was time-consuming. Nurses working in similar situations appear to come together and state that their professional expectation of each other is to offer the 'gift' of emotion work, recognising it takes time and effort (Bolton 2000). The acknowledgment and acceptance of these framing rules appears to reduce some of the emotional labour experienced by them when offering the 'gift'.

Circle of Care

As identified in the previous paragraphs, emotional care, particularly emotional support, is time-consuming, but midwives are not usually alone in their provision of support. In chapter 2, all those who may be involved in offering emotional support to women on their journey to motherhood was discussed. It was recognised that the family, particularly the father of the baby or the partner of the woman, was a significant participator in this.

The midwives in my study described their interactions with other family members when identifying their emotional support of women. They described what one of them labelled a 'circle of care'. This circle of care could consist of the midwife and father or other members of the family, but could also involve the midwife and other health professionals. The members of the 'circle of care' were dependant on the available support from family and friends and the needs of the women.

Family members, as part of this circle of care, assisted the midwives in their showing care or offering support to the women, but they also, at times, needed support themselves from the midwives. The support offered to the partners of the women varied, depending on the midwives' perception of their need. Gina offered information and activities for the partner at quite a stressful time. She said,

> "I said you don't need to do anything, if she has the baby before anybody gets to the house you don't need to do anything, just lift the baby to her abdomen and dry the baby off and use that towel and then throw it away and get another towel to wrap the baby in".

Gina continued to offer reassurance and support to the woman's husband until the paramedics arrived; she then also offered guidance to them.

Fiona also recognised the importance of the emotional support that could be offered by the partner or other members of the family and explained she organised her visits to facilitate their being at the woman's home at the same time. She said,

> "I was also able to support him as well; that's the other issue, that emotional support is not just for women, because if you can emotionally support the partner, the mum or whoever the person is likely to be, they are then empowered to support the women".

Whilst other midwives also recognised the importance of a family member, particularly the partner's support through their non-verbal communication, this did not always reduce their workload. This can be seen in the statement above by Fiona, but Betty and Diane identify that it caused them certain levels of stress and emotion work.

Betty acknowledged that the husband could support her and his wife, which was especially important given their particular struggles with communication. She said,

> "Using a few minutes to explain to him to get him to understand and be reassured, so when I'm telling her when she looked at him she could see a happy face, a relaxed face which meant it could reassure her".

Recognising how helpful it was to have the husband involved, albeit only minimally, reduced Betty's emotion work but she was concerned about putting the woman first. Betty found herself torn between explaining information to the husband first so he could support his wife, and attempting to explain more slowly to both of them together, which would take longer to reduce the concern. She said,

> "But normally one would think it better to talk to the lady, but if she is sat there and he is sat there and not knowing what is being said and he is worried, she is going to look to him and see a worried face".

As can be seen from these midwives, families can offer support to both the woman and midwife, but they also need support to fulfil this role.

There are also times when members of the family actually increase the emotional care needed by women. For Carol, the family were quite negative about breast-feeding, which midwives are guided to encourage.

> "Her family weren't particularly pro- breast feeding, they were quite derogatory about breast feeding".

This negativity led to ambivalence in the woman and an increased her need for support from Carol.

As indicated, the circle of care could involve family and friends or other health professionals. All the midwives in my study described other professionals playing a part in this circle of care for the women, and some talked of the emotional support they received from this circle too. Betty said,

> "Umm I work in a very good team anyway where we all support each other" and "the support basically came from the Health Visitor and the GP because we had formed a little circle around this lady; whoever saw her next would talk to the other two".

'Unique Normality'

Supportive midwifery practices are providing an environment that focuses on the normality of motherhood, including the birth, reduced fear and increased confidence, control and trust (Rhodes 1995, Edwards 2000, Kirkham 2000, NICE 2004, ICM 2006). There appears, though, to be some lack of clarity over the term "normal". Normal behaviour in psychology has been much debated and a number of theories have arisen (Barker 2007). Similarly, the definition of 'normal birth' in midwifery has also caused some debate. Midwifery is one of the few healthcare professions whose focus is on normality – the normality of birth. Most healthcare professionals focus on abnormality: distress, deviance, dysfunction or dangerous behaviours.

Despite the emphasis from midwifery bodies and government initiatives to promote 'normal birth', this remains problematic within our society. Not only are there problems with a clear definition for midwives to work with, but there are also other cultural factors that need to be taken into account. These factors include the risk-aversive, litigious culture (Fraser and Cooper 2003, McGuinness 2006) but also the women who are giving birth have expectations from their mothers of medical intervention (Skinner 2005). This becomes even more problematic when women might choose to have a caesarean, rather than a vaginal birth, when there is no medical necessity (Fraser and Cooper 2003). There is actually no conclusive evidence to support what normal birth is or when it should occur (Fraser and Cooper 2003, Phipps 2005).

'Unique normality' (Downe 2006) may address both the specialness of each woman and the normality of their experience. This can be achieved by avoiding rigid rules and developing authentic respectful relationships between midwives and the women and families they care for (Downe 2006). Skinner (2005) would support Downe's way forward and she goes on to suggest that to promote normal birth, midwives need to fit midwifery services to women and not fit women to the midwifery services.

John and Parsons (2006), who conducted their study in the UK, considered the emotion work of midwives and their findings link with the concept of normality. In their study they found four interlinking themes, which were 'presentation of self, establishing rapport and personal and professional emotion', 'pulling the shutter down' from the midwives and 'perceptions of shadow work' and 'the maintenance of normality' from the mothers. The maintenance of normality was important for the mother's wellbeing and the midwives attempted to achieve this by using emotion work to develop a rapport with them.

Rapport for those spoken with and observed by John and Parsons (2006: 268) was expressed as "basic care, touch, facial encouragement, chit- chat and sharing part of themselves". These can be seen as very similar approaches to those used in relationship development to offer emotional support for the midwives in my study and have already been discussed in this chapter.

John and Parsons' (2006) study provided the women's perspective on the importance of being treated as if they were normal and the midwives behaving as if they were having normal conversations. The midwives in their study also identified that they were trying to ensure the whole experience was normal for the women. The experience of being 'normal' appears to have a duality of meaning within midwifery, in that the midwives appear to try to facilitate a 'normal birth' and the experience of 'being normal' also appears to mean the woman not being distressed, or believing that there is anything wrong with her. They appear to use both meanings of normal and attempt to achieve both types of normality to facilitate the women gaining comfort (Morse et al 1994).

The midwives in my study also identified the need to allow the women to have a sense of normality to create comfort in them. They felt it was important that the women should feel that their experiences were normal and the midwives also tried to encourage the women to believe that their births were normal. This was demonstrated in several of the midwives' descriptions. Through their close relationships, the midwives can be seen to be attempting to facilitate a feeling of comfort in the woman by providing her with recognition that her perceptions of her experiences were understandable and not a sign of deviance or disorder.

Fiona believed there were a lot of common thoughts and feelings amongst new mothers, which allowed her to say to the woman that it was fine to feel the way she did. She also said it was incredibly reassuring to the woman to be told there is nothing wrong. Betty also believed that it was important for women, when they are vulnerable, such as when they are pregnant or the early days after birth, to feel normal. Likewise Carol said, *"I think really we need to make them feel they are normal and are not abnormal in any way; that this is normal"*.

It is again difficult to know if the midwives held the belief that they should encourage the sense of normality because they are led to do so by government guidelines or whether there is another ideological reason for this. The 'with woman' ideology supports the belief that becoming a mother is a normal process, not a medical condition requiring intervention. This is an ideological standpoint that is being increasingly promoted by government, as well as midwives (NSF – DoH 2004).

As already stated, supportive midwifery practices include providing an environment that focuses on the normality of motherhood (including the birth), reduced fear and increased confidence, control and trust (Rhodes 1995, Edwards 2000, Kirkham 2000, NICE 2003, ICM 2006). All the midwives in my study demonstrated their focus on normality, despite at times struggling with the women's perception that their experience was not normal. For example, Carol said, *"I don't know why she found it traumatic; it was a normal birth"*.

When it was recognised that the women did not feel their experiences to be normal, the midwives endeavoured to persuade the women that they were. Where this was not achieved, this became, for some, a trigger to offering emotional support and created emotion work for the midwife. All the midwives in my study could also be seen to be trying to facilitate reduced fear, increased confidence, control and trust as recommended by their professional body, government guidelines and research evidence (Rhodes 1995, Edwards 2000, Kirkham 2000, NICE 2003, ICM 2006) through their intimate midwife-woman relationship.

Summary

The core term for what midwives do is care (NMC 2008, ICM 2006). This is enacted through the midwife-woman relationship, but it is considered difficult to achieve in the current culture of opposing ideologies (Hunter 2004) and NHS management (Kirkham 1999) and this will be discussed in detail in chapter 5. What midwives do is provide care to facilitate women's transition to motherhood safely; this is a skilful and complex role. This can be seen through the literature and the descriptions from the midwives. The descriptions of the midwives in my study also demonstrate that, for them, there are other elements to this already acknowledged skilful and complex role.

The midwives demonstrate that emotional support is provided through this caring relationship, but the emotionally supportive midwifery relationship is special. It is more intimate and has closer physical proximity than other therapeutic relationships. This relationship is developed and maintained through skilful communication. The midwives described their communication skills, both non-verbal and verbal. Non-verbally they listened, gained eye contact and sensitively touched women in accordance with their perceived need. Despite these descriptions there is evidence in the literature that, when midwives believe they are doing this, they are actually focused on other things (Lomax and Robinson 1996) and not actively listening (Egan 1977). The midwives in my study, in their descriptions, appear to be undertaking these other tasks in a supportive manner; it could therefore be labelled emotional care.

The midwives managed situations to provide this extra support, by making time and visiting the women at home, which they believed facilitated a more relaxed environment where women felt more in control. Control and choice, advocated by professional bodies (ICM 2006) and government (DoH 1993), was further enhanced by the midwives' verbal skills and information- giving. This is another area of contention in the literature, as it has been found that midwives do not always give all the information to women to enable them to make complete, informed decisions. The protective steering identified by Levy (1999d), could also be seen in the midwives in my findings. It was unclear whether the midwives in my study were consciously using protective steering to emotionally support the women, but they clearly identified moderating and managing the information they gave and appeared to believe they were doing what was best for the women.

Emotionally supportive qualities appear to be listening, touch, being respectful, acceptance and giving clear information (Schuiling and Sampselle 1999, Edwards 2000, Morse 2000). These should be undertaken, whatever the midwifery task may be, such as clinical examinations, if the aim is to offer comfort (Morse 2000). Supportive midwifery practices include providing an environment that focuses on the normality of motherhood (including the birth), reduced fear, and increased confidence, control and trust (Rhodes 1995, Edwards 2000, Kirkham 2000, NICE 2003, ICM 2006). All of these attitudes and behaviours can be seen in the midwives in my study when providing emotional care but there are also additional elements that they describe. These are the circle of care, home visiting, giving time, the use of self, and continuity of individual relationships.

Essentially, the phenomenon of giving emotional support to women becoming mothers can most usefully and simply be labelled a type of showing care; it is part of emotional care. This care is enacted by the midwives through the extensive use of their communication skills, as can be seen in other therapeutic relationships. The relationship between midwives and women, though, can be considered more intimate in nature due to physical and personal proximity. Midwives provide this care within a circle – the circle of care, which involves other professionals and the woman's family. As the midwives provide this care, they appear to seek to promote feelings of comfort and control in the women, in what can seem like a time of inner insecurity, lack of control and emotional turmoil.

This is to facilitate their journey to motherhood, as emotional distress at this time can have long- term consequences, such as postnatal depression.

CHAPTER FIVE

WHAT ARE THE EXPERIENCES OF MIDWIVES GIVING EMOTIONAL SUPPORT?

Introduction

There has been increased interest from midwifery researchers in the area of emotions, especially emotional labour and emotion work, leading to a number of recent publications. Despite this, there remains a limited description of midwives' experiences of offering emotional support or care for women becoming mothers. The early work of Oakley (1988, 1992) and the study by Hildingsson and Häggström (1999) on supporting women is, though, a useful starting point. The research on emotion work, by Hunter and colleagues, has further opened up the area to scrutiny. Leading on from these publications, the study undertaken by myself is the core study used here to explore the experiences of midwives offering emotional support to women on their journey to motherhood.

Ann Oakley undertook sociological research, related to social support and motherhood, for over twenty five years and has published numerous journal articles and books in the area. These were mostly based on the Social Support and Pregnancy Outcomes (SSPO) Study. For this study, social support was defined as "the provision of a non-judgemental listening ear, discussing with women their pregnancy needs, giving information when asked to, and carrying out referrals when appropriate to other health and welfare professionals and voluntary and statutory agencies" (Oakley 1992: 144). Oakley's book "Social Support and Motherhood" in 1992 brought together some of her understanding of both the area and how to research it. Her work, along with her colleagues, recognises the importance of the culture in which motherhood occurs and the impact of social support on the health of mothers and babies. The SSPO demonstrates that social support is effective, appropriate and safe for high risk mothers.

Hildingsson and Häggström undertook a significant study in 1999. This foundational piece of research was undertaken in Sweden. Hildingsson and Häggström explored the experiences of seven midwives supporting women during pregnancy. They used a hermeneutic phenomenological approach, which allowed them to gain some insight into how midwives fulfilled their supportive role. Their findings, as with complementary studies by Bondas and Eriksson (2001) and Barclay et al (1997) of women's experiences, may be different to the experiences of midwives in the UK, due to cultural differences, but they could offer some valuable insights.

Hildingsson and Häggström (1999) found that the midwives in their study took on a role of the 'good mother' which, for them, was both exhausting and time-consuming, but also joyful. As part of this role, the midwives were said to encourage autonomy whilst offering advocacy. They also found, in contrast, the role of 'good mother' played by the midwives could also restrict autonomy and integrity, which is advocated within midwifery education. It also led midwives to admonish the women at times.

Fifteen subcategories were found and they were organised into four themes. The four themes were 'caring actions based on ethical reflections and situational insights', 'prospective fathers', 'involvement and advocacy' and 'reflective evaluation of work'.

Caring actions, based on ethical reflections and situational insights, involved a wish to be 'good'; the midwives wanted to do their best for the women. It is interesting that both the mothers and midwives wanted to achieve something they label as 'good', the 'good mother', the 'good midwife'. The midwives, in this study and incorporated into this theme, verbalised their personal responsibilities and the ethical demands on them (Hildingsson and Häggström's 1999). Alongside this they respected the woman's autonomy and supported her right to make informed choices. To achieve being a 'good midwife', to address the ethical demands and support autonomy, the midwives gained knowledge about the women's situations and their support needs.

Prospective fathers did appear in the interview transcripts, but not in an explicit manner; the scripts needed to be searched to find their presence. The theme of involvement and advocacy involved recognition that the midwives held a professional, as well as personal, role in their support of the women. They used both professional and personal time to provide the care they felt was needed. Their advocacy role also had a number of parts. They advocated for the rights of the baby to receive good care; likewise the woman and the baby's father. Alongside this, they advocated for the woman and the baby's father by empowering them to make choices.

In their evaluative reflections of their support of the women, the midwives identified that it was an important task to facilitate the growth and development of the women. They also reflected on the opportunities to achieve job satisfaction and how limited these were. The workload was suggested to be burdensome and the midwives felt undervalued, but also found it rewarding and joyful (Hildingsson and Häggström 1999).

This study by Hildingsson and Häggström (1999) was the only one, at this time, that focused specifically on midwives' experiences of supporting women becoming mothers, but others offer valuable insights into how midwives experience offering emotionally supportive care. John and Parsons' study (2006) focused on the emotion work of midwives and Bone's study (2009), which focused on the care- deficit in maternity units in the US, offer some understanding.

John and Parsons (2006) conducted their study in the UK with midwives and women on a delivery suite in a low- risk, obstetric unit. They used an ethnographic approach, observing and interviewing ten midwives and the women they were working with. Four interlinking themes were identified, which were labelled 'presentation of self, establishing rapport and personal and professional emotion' and 'pulling the shutter down' from the midwives and 'perceptions of shadow work' and 'the maintenance of normality' from the mothers.

Hildingsson and Häggström's (1999) and John and Parsons' (2006) studies revealed an attempt by the midwives to develop rapport. This was expressed, by the midwives Hildingsson and Häggström interviewed, as getting to know the woman's situation and needs. Rapport for those spoken with and observed by John and Parsons (2006: 268) was expressed as "basic care, touch, facial encouragement, chit- chat and sharing part of themselves".

Another more recent study conducted in the US also had some similar findings (Bone 2009). Although it was undertaken with nurses, they were fulfilling what would be considered a midwifery role on a labour ward in the UK. As part of this study, the nurses were asked to describe how they provided emotional support. The nurses identified "'ways of being, doing and knowing', that could be considered therapeutic emotional labour" (Bone 2009: 59). According to Bone (2009: 60), these ways of being, doing and knowing are "intuitive, relational, experiential and situated".

Bone found that it was difficult for the nurses to distinguish between emotional support and just chatting. Chatting was also identified as a technique for offering emotional support, by John and Parsons (2006) in their study. The nurses described their activities in a way that minimised the value attached to them, which could be seen to devalue emotional support, by frequently using the term 'just' (Bone 2009). Emotional support appeared to be incidental to other activities, such as measurement and documentation, particularly in Bone's study, but the 'chatting' in John and Parsons' study can be viewed in a similar way.

The nurses Bone interviewed, described 'being there' and listening as helpful in emotional support, but explained that it was more about how things were done, rather than a distinct activity, that facilitated calm or relaxed behaviour in the women. This had already been highlighted by Morse (1994) in her study on providing comfort. The nurses also described using their intuition, perceptiveness or a sixth sense to guide them. Hildingsson and Häggström (1999: 85), like Bone (2009), described midwives using intuition or some other kind of interpretative tool as "they heard something between the words the woman said". This use of self can be seen to make the relationship between midwife and women more intimate.

The literature available suggests that supporting women on their journey to motherhood is stressful, exhausting and undervalued and leads to emotion work (Hildingsson and Häggström 1999, John and Parsons 2006, Bone 2009). Hunter and colleagues have, throughout the last decade, conducted a number of studies exploring this emotion work, which is briefly considered in this chapter, but more fully considered in chapter 6. To understand the emotional support of women on their journey to motherhood, it is perhaps best to explore it as an unfurling process, in line with my descriptive phenomenological study of how midwives experience offering emotional support to women on their journey to motherhood. This process starts with how midwives come to be offering emotional support and moves on initially to the culture in which this occurs and then to some of the struggles they experience along the way.

Decision making

The midwives in John and Parsons' study (2006) and the nurses in Bone's study (2009) appeared to perceive emotional support as part of their regular care for women. In contrast, the midwives in Hildingsson and Häggström's (1999) study appeared to put extra effort into emotionally caring for women. This was also the case in my study. The judgement to offer emotionally supportive care for these midwives was not an easy one to make. They appeared to be impeded by their professional belief that family or friends should offer emotional support, which weighted the decision against showing this type of care. Alongside this was the belief that not all women needed emotional support. When there needed to be a movement towards providing emotional care the midwives, within what appeared to be a technical medical focus, moved to a more emotional focus.

To allow themselves to offer emotional care, the midwives gave themselves reasons, such as that the woman had had a traumatic birth, physical illness or a lack of social support. If the midwife could not find a suitable reason like this, they provided themselves with the justification that the woman probably had 'underlying issues'. As explained by one of the midwives in my study,

> "Pregnancy and birth can bring back ghosts from the past that you didn't even realise were there".

As indicated by one midwife, Fiona, it was felt that not all women need emotional support,

> "A person who is very confident and outspoken and in which case you won't need emotional support".

Despite this, it was recognised by the midwives in this study that it is difficult to assess if women will need this type of care. As highlighted by Emily, it was difficult to assess who would need extra support, as the woman she described was from a good socio-economic background with family support, but she needed extended support and visiting.

This decision to offer emotional support was also influenced by what the midwives identified as a 'moment of realisation'. The midwives stated that there is a moment of realisation when the woman is more vulnerable. In their descriptions, this realisation could occur during pregnancy, during the birth or in the days after the birth, which is upheld by previous literature (Barclay et al 1997, Cronin 2003). This indicates that all women may need emotional support, at some stage, during their journey to motherhood.

The National Service Framework ((NSF) DoH 2004) offers a vision for maternity care which promotes a flexible and individualised service for the journey through pregnancy and motherhood, with a particular focus on those women who are disadvantaged or vulnerable. Whilst the midwives would appear to agree that flexible, individualised care is important, they do not appear to wholly agree that there is a need to focus on the disadvantaged and vulnerable. Some suggest, along with my findings, that all women need support as, regardless of which socio-economic group they are in, there will be differing but similarly problematic struggles with becoming a mother in the current social climate (Cattrell et al 2005).

The suggestion, that not all women need emotionally supportive care from midwives, was also demonstrated in my study in the descriptions the midwives gave of when they provided this type of care. Each situation was unique, but the midwives felt the need to describe these in detail, which could lead to the conclusion that midwives need to have a justification for offering this special or extra care. This need for justification could be considered to be part of the culture, either of midwifery within the local environment, or more generally. Another element that appears to run through the descriptions in my study is that the midwives were concerned for the emotional well-being of mother and baby.

All the midwives, who described their emotional support in my study, had concerns about the woman and identified her as either already being emotionally distressed, or at risk of becoming so. Midwives could therefore be seen to be offering emotionally supportive care to reduce or ameliorate both emotional distress and the risk of it.

In my study, the midwives within their regular, professional, caring activities appeared to weigh up the decision whether to emphasise emotionally supportive care. As part of this weighing up, they assessed initially if the women had any specific problems and then if they had had a normal birth, or had had some scope for making choices through their journey to motherhood.

The midwives appeared to desire to offer emotional support, as demonstrated by their willingness to provide a reason, such as 'underlying causes', when no other reason was easily available but, despite this, they appeared to need to provide a justification for giving this type of care.

Other literature available, in contrast, indicates that all women need emotional support (DoH 2004, ICM 2006, Page and McCandlish 2006). The same literature also encourages the midwife to support the woman's family. As already stated, the NSF (DoH 2004) identifies that there are some women with greater need of emotional support, in particular those who are socially disadvantaged. Despite this, much of the midwifery literature appears to guide midwives to develop technical, biomedical care (DoH 1997, 1998, 2000, Way 2000, NICE 2003, 2006, Johnson and Taylor 2006).

The need to provide a justification for the midwives in my study may be due to the extra resources required to provide emotional support. For them, as well as the midwives in Hildingsson and Häggström's study (1999), providing emotional support required extra activities and time.

The movement towards a decision to offer emotional support, as identified in my study, does not appear to occur in other studies, such as Bolton's (2000) or Bone's study (2009), where it was indicated by their participants that emotional support is given during regular activities. It does need to be acknowledged, though, that the midwives in my study and similarly in Hildingsson and Häggström's study (1999), were community midwives and they had the autonomy to manage their provision of care, which may not have been available to those working in a ward environment, such the participants of Bolton's and Bone's studies.

Emotional support appeared to be incidental, in comparison to other activities such as measurement and documentation, for the midwives in the study by Bone (2009), but this was not found in the midwives in this or Hildingsson and Häggström's studies (1999). It can, though, be seen that these other technical tasks were of priority for them. Emotional support, for the midwives in the studies of Bone (2009) and John and Parsons (2006), was identified in how things were done, rather than in a distinct activity to facilitate calm or relaxed behaviour in the women. Despite the midwives in this study and Hildingsson and Häggström's study (1999) identifying specific activities to undertake emotional support, this approach to regular care could also be seen in their findings.

It can be seen that community midwives go through some sort of decision-making process to decide whether to undertake the extra activity of providing emotional support to women on their journey to motherhood, which may not be the situation for those working in institutions. Hunter (2004, 2005), in her exploration of emotion work, clearly identified these two environments as adhering to differing ideologies. She suggests that midwives who work in institutions adhere to a 'with institute' ideology, whereas midwives working in the community work within a 'with woman' ideology.

The ideology to which a midwife adheres can be seen to be influential to the way in which they work. This ideology is closely linked to the culture within which people work. The generally prevailing ideologies within Western society were discussed in chapter 1. The ideology explored by Hunter (2004, 2005) was more specific to midwifery as underlying the professions culture.

Culture

Historical context

The professional role of midwives, along with the culture in which they work, has changed over the years and, in fact, it was only in the twentieth century that midwives gained the status of being professionals. Midwives as autonomous professionals developed due, in part, to increasing medicalisation and acknowledged experts managing and taking control of (expert-led) childbirth. Between the First and Second World Wars, in the 1920s and 1930s, there was a focus on the risk for mother and baby, which led to the perceived need for doctors to be involved in childbirth. The involvement of doctors led to increased hospitalisation of women and encouraged an expert-led approach to maternity care (Littlewood and McHugh 1997). Midwives were an intrinsic part of these developments and medicalisation influenced their journey to professionalism. It has been an eventful process, influenced by social need, politics and religion.

There is evidence of wise women assisting other women in childbirth for as long as documentation has been available, reaching back to what may be considered the beginnings of civilisation in Mesopotamia. Religious doctrine has had implications for those supporting women in childbirth, in Christian or Jewish societies, for two reasons. Firstly, it was considered by those of faith that women, for leading men to sin, were condemned to suffer great pain in childbirth. Secondly, women were viewed as more susceptible to evil. For orthodox followers, this put the wise women, caring for women in childbirth, in a precarious position, as both midwives and mothers were already seen as tainted by original sin and therefore at high risk of demonic possession. The Catholic Church was powerful in Europe in the 15th century, which led to a wide acceptance of the Malleus Malificarum (1486), which identified midwives as likely candidates as witches (Littlewood and McHugh 1997). The oppression perceived by some prominent midwives (Kirkham 2000) may have its early roots here in religious texts.

In the Middle Ages, midwives continued to carry out the role of caring for women in childbirth. They had no training, were mostly illiterate, as were most of the population, and clearly took the role of midwife; with women. These midwives also had a religious role, in that part of their job was to baptise sickly babies so that their souls would not be lost. In 1513 Eucharius Rosslin (a doctor) wrote a book for midwives called The Rose Garden of Pregnant Women and Midwives. Despite this book being written by a man, for midwives and women, doctors or males were virtually never admitted to the room of a labouring woman. Rosslin's book stated that the midwife's role is to "instruct and comfort the party" (Rhodes 1995: 15). Comfort was achieved by offering good food and drink, expressing sweet words and gentle stroking.

The central figure in midwifery in the 18th century was William Smellie, who became known as the Master of British Midwifery. He began teaching midwifery to both men and women, in separate classes, in 1741. He wrote books to facilitate the learning of his students: in 1742 'A course of lectures upon midwifery' and in 1752 'A treatise on the theory and practice of midwifery'. His male midwives were trained to use instruments, such as forceps, and dealt with difficult births, whereas the female midwives helped women with normal births. Whereas previously the labour room was reserved for women, this changed with the training of male midwives. The male midwives were called in when the female midwives were having problems. This can be seen to have driven a wedge between the sexes and sometimes created antagonism in the birthing room (Rhodes 1995). There was still a strong Christian ethos in British society and this identified that childbirth facilitated the way to salvation for women, as long as they retained a subordinate position to men (Littlewood and McHugh 1997).

In the early 19th century there was recognition of the need to organise and structure medicine. At this stage, women were not allowed to become doctors and these "gentlemen of enlarged academic education" (Rhodes 1995: 85) were advised not be involved in the labouring of women. Seventeen acts of parliament were enacted between 1840 and 1858 in an attempt to regulate and structure medicine, but it was not until 1886 that midwifery (now known as obstetrics) was included as an area of study for doctors (Rhodes 1995).

Maternal and infant deaths were high in the 19th century, with the poor being particularly at risk. This became a significant problem when the government was seeking men to fight in the Boer War and found few fit enough to provide a good army. This led to legislation relating to childbirth (Littlewood and McHugh 1997). Alongside this there was pressure from obstetricians, who called for the training and regulation of midwives to be in the same manner as doctors. Educated, middle- and upper- class midwives were quick to take up this challenge, with many completing the voluntary London Obstetrics Society examination prior to compulsory training commencing (Rhodes 1995). This was the foundation for the development of midwifery as a profession in the 20th century.

Through the centuries it can be seen that women have been subordinated and there appears to have been some fear attached to them, particularly those who assisted in childbirth, leading to the suggestion they may be witches. It might also be suggested that, despite professionalising midwifery and childbirth being considered a way to improve care, it is another way of controlling feared women.

In 1902, in England, the government passed the first Midwives Act, which separated two of the main roles of the wise women, that of laying out dead people and assisting in childbirth. The Act said the same person should not undertake both these roles (Littlewood and McHugh 1997). It may also be seen as the start of men and medicine taking over what was, until then, a woman's domain (Mander and Reid 2002). The Act also involved the setting up of a Central Midwives Board in England and Wales; registration with the board was necessary in order to practice as a midwife. It can be seen that gone were the days of the wise women or, as they were known at the time, the handy women. It has been suggested that women who came from the middle and upper classes were in league with their male counterparts, the doctors, to remove competition and establish their place as professionals (Leap and Hunter 1993).

The Central Midwives Board set standards for entry to the midwives' register, including training and certification, along with guidelines for removal from the register. The Midwives, who had supported this introduction, found that as well as removing the competition of the handy women, who had been used as the scapegoat for the high maternal mortality rate (Leap and Hunter 1993), they also had their own scope of practice limited. These professional midwives were now only allowed to work with women who were experiencing 'normal' childbirth; they had to call a doctor if there were any complications (Mander and Reid 2002).

The third Midwives Act was implemented in 1926. This saw a formalisation of the teaching of midwives, along with an identified midwife teachers' certificate and the fining of unregistered people for attending births, unless it was an emergency situation (Leap and Hunter 1993). The start of the medicalisation of births had already begun but was increasing in momentum, with 15% of births occurring in institutions in 1927, increasing to 24% by 1932 and 45% by 1944 (Leap and Hunter 1993). This had increased to 64% by 1952 (Rhodes 1995).

The founding of the College of Midwives, which set the training and standards for midwives, occurred in 1933. They focused on the provision of antenatal care and more expert intervention in childbirth. Antenatal care, or pre-maternity care, proliferated at this time with Ballantyne, an obstetrician, laying down that the aims of this care should include: "removal of dread, reduce discomfort, treating syphilis and toxaemia early, increase normal pregnancies and labours, reduce still births, and reduce maternal mortality" (Rhodes 1995: 123). This was particularly interesting due to its emphasis on psychological, as well as physical, well-being.

The National Health Service was introduced in 1948 and midwifery services were included in this. By the 1960's there was a call for all births to be in hospital and in the 1970's and '80's, with increasing medical interventions available and consumer- led health care, this gained momentum (Peel Report 1970, Court Report 1976, Welburn 1980 cited in Littlewood and McHugh 1997).

As can be seen, midwifery has a long history, but as a profession most development was in the 20th century. The 20th century saw huge changes in the care of women in their transition to motherhood, through the assuming of professional status by midwives and the medical interventions in childbirth. With medical developments, such as antibiotics and blood transfusions, mortality rates decreased. This may be the reason women increasingly wanted to give birth in hospital. They saw hospitals as safer than their own homes, showing a cultural change in childbirth (Rhodes 1995).

Since the 1950s the risk of death during childbirth has decreased and routine processes have been developed to care for women in pregnancy, labour and the early postnatal days. Professional midwives and obstetricians are now taking women through these processes and increasingly using technological screening of both mother and baby. During this period "the woman's whole life changes immeasurably", due in part to great mental and emotional upheavals, after giving birth to a baby (Rhodes 1995: 176). A lack of recognition of these emotional and psychological factors may have led to recent figures, which suggest most maternal deaths in the UK are due to mental health and psychological problems (Drift 2004).

Some have suggested that the emotional or psychological problems experienced by women may be influenced by the medicalisation and the medical power base which puts women and midwives in an oppressive position (Mander and Reid 2002, Littlewood and McHugh 1997). Despite the publication of the Winterton Report in 1992 and Changing Childbirth in 1993 (DoH 1993), advocating a 'woman-centred' approach within midwifery, there are those who would suggest that this appears to be mostly rhetorical (Mander and Reid 2002).

In 1991 The Winterton Committee produced its report on its investigation of maternity services (Tew 1998). The report recommended continuity of care and carer (which they believed was best undertaken by midwives) and that women should be given choices related to their care, allowing them to feel in control. The Royal College of Midwives, although acknowledging and supporting the desires of women, stipulated that midwives should be allowed to overrule these desires if they thought it necessary through their professional knowledge and skills (Tew 1998).

In response to the Winterton Report, the Department of Health set up an Expert Maternity Group to consider how the wide-ranging recommendations could be put into practice. This group produced a report in 1993 called

'Changing Childbirth' (DoH 1993) and its main recommendations are worth considering here.

The key principles of maternity care, identified in the Changing Childbirth report, were that women should be the focus of maternity care: that it should be women-centred. Maternity services should be easily accessible to all women and they should be involved in the development and planning of their care (Henderson and Jones 1997). The report stipulates that women should know who is going to support them in labour and who the lead professional is in planning their care. Women should have the right to clear, unbiased information. Obstetricians' skills should be used for complicated births, but care should be more community- orientated and practice should be evidence-based. The Royal College of Obstetricians were unhappy with a couple of elements of this report. These concerns centred on the implications that they would not have jurisdiction over normal births and that home births were recognised as a safe alternative to hospital births (Henderson and Jones 1997).

This brief overview of the development of midwifery care, up to the late twentieth century, shows the cultural movements. Initially, a 'with woman' ideology appears to have been underlying care, as handywomen had little scientific knowledge and supported women with their experiential knowledge. The scientific developments in medicine fuelled a move for women to be supported using a medical approach, to reduce mortality and morbidity rates associated with motherhood. The beginning of the twentieth century saw the institutionalisation of maternal care and the professionalisation of midwives, which could be considered the foundation of the 'with institution' or 'with profession' ideology. The Winterton report and changing childbirth report appeared to have encouraged, for some, maternal care to swing back towards a more 'with woman' ideology. There were, though, many more influencing factors to affect the ideological underpinning of midwifery.

Alongside the influential maternity-focused reports, the 1990's saw massive changes in the structure of the National Health Service, which started with the publication of the white paper 'The New NHS – Modern and Dependable' (DoH 1997). This identified the need for patient-centred care and aimed to exchange the internal market, developed by Margaret Thatcher's conservative government, for a more integrated approach. This can be seen to lead to the establishment of clinical governance and quality, evidence-based care through the publication of 'A First Class

Service' (DoH 1998). Introduction of bodies, such as the National Institute of Clinical Excellence (NICE) and structures such as the National Service Frameworks (NSF), were developed to ensure evidence-based, quality care was accessible by all, regardless of where they lived.

Recent Guidance

The National Service Framework (NSF) for Children, Young People and Maternity Services in England was published by the Department of Health in 2004. In Standard 11 of this NSF, it clearly states that the psychological and emotional needs of the mother should be assessed and care provided through a multidisciplinary, team-based approach. NICE published guidelines for antenatal care in 2003 and followed this up with guidelines for postnatal care in 2006. The antenatal guidelines, whilst stating the need to address women's anxieties promptly, do not encourage screening for psychiatric illness in the antenatal period, in order to predict postnatal mental health problems, as there is no evidence that this is effective. They do, though, clearly state that if the woman has had previous mental illness, she should be referred for specialist assessment (Sidebotham 2004). Further guidelines have been issued by NICE on antenatal care (2008) and they have produced guidance on perinatal mental health (NICE 2007). These documents uphold the previous guidance that women should be asked about previous personal or family mental health problems at their booking appointment with the midwife. The NICE guidance (2007, 2008) also recommends that for those women identified as at risk there should be clear plans in place and specialist support available. Despite local service developments to implement these recommendations Rowan et al (2010) found that although women were being screened at the booking appointment services were fragmented and liaison between professional groups was limited.

The introduction of the NSF for maternity matters and the NICE guidance appear to have made the psychological and emotional needs of women higher profile but the majority of their guidance refers what could be labelled medical-technical care.

Despite the extensive guidance on medical-technical care, there has been reference throughout the centuries to the need for those caring for women becoming mothers to be kind, offering soothing words and reducing distress. Unfortunately, with the progression of the professionalisation of midwifery and the medicalisation of childbirth, it is suggested that maternal emotional distress has increased (Littlewood and McHugh 1997), perhaps indicating that this kind caring is not occurring.

Considering current midwifery educational texts, the development of the profession, legislation and policy, it can be agreed that midwives assist women during pregnancy, birth and the early days after the birth of the baby. How this is undertaken is now guided by government bodies through legislation and policy. The primary guiding policies at the present time are The National Service Framework (NSF) for Children, Young People and Maternity Services (DoH 2004), Antenatal Care (NICE 2003, 2008) and Routine postnatal care of women and babies (NICE 2006).

The NSF (DoH 2004) offers a vision for maternity care which promotes a flexible and individualised service for the journey through pregnancy and motherhood, with a particular focus on those women who are disadvantaged or vulnerable. Whilst midwives would appear to agree that flexible, individualised care is important, they do not appear to wholly agree that there is a need to focus on the disadvantaged and vulnerable. Some suggest that all women need support as, regardless of which socio-economic group they are in, there will be differing but similarly problematic struggles with becoming a mother in the current social climate (Cattrell et al 2005).

The NSF (DoH 2004) also states that women should be 'supported' and 'encouraged' to have as 'normal' a pregnancy and birth as possible. Both midwifery and obstetric care should be based on evidence of good outcomes, clinically and psychologically, whilst putting equal emphasis on preparation for parenthood. This could be seen to have, unsurprisingly, a high correlation to the NICE antenatal (2003, 2008) and postnatal care (2006) guidelines, with their focus on women-centred care and informed decision-making. Despite this similar philosophical stance, a more detailed reading of the guidelines could lead the midwife to believe they should focus on screening and examination in the antenatal period and information- giving in the postnatal period.

The role of the midwife has developed since the beginning of civilisation. It has mostly been the role of women to support others in childbirth and over the centuries they have faced extensive subordination. This may still influence both women and midwives, in the current society. Despite this subordination midwives have gained professional status, but this appears to have created a further dilemma for midwives in how they view themselves and their role.

Philosophy of care

Rather than adhering to implicit ideological demands it could be suggested that an agreed philosophy of care is adopted. There are those who suggest that the philosophy of care a midwife should adhere to is being ‘with woman’, offering understanding, kindness and comfort (Leap and Hunter 1993, Rhodes 1995, Kirkham 2000, Page and McCandlish 2006). Others imply that the focus, or philosophical underpinning a midwife should have, is a professional one, with a greater emphasis on biological and technical care (DoH 1997, 1998, 2000, NICE 2003, 2006). There are, though, those who recommend a mixture of the two approaches (DoH 2004, ICM 2006). The most powerful of the influences on the role of a midwife could be seen to be government-funded sources (NICE, DoH, NHS) who employ most midwives. This could lead midwives to believe that the professional approach should be adopted; this would then influence how they behave and what they do.

The development of midwifery as a profession was not a smooth, uneventful, process. Events, such as the Midwives Acts and policy development, influence the midwifery culture experienced by midwives today. The Midwives Acts were introduced to develop a trained and disciplined profession, where the midwives’ first loyalty would now be to their profession, rather than to the women for whom they cared (Kirkham 1999). The introduction of the National Health Service (NHS) led to an increase in midwives and an increase in the power which the organisational system had over them. Both the NHS and language used can be seen as male engendered, forming an early wedge between ‘being with women’ and ‘being professional’ (Kirkham 1999). The issue of patriarchy in health and caring has been raised by a number of other writers (Morrison 1992, Littlewood and McHugh 1997). In her review of the literature, Kirkham (1999) acknowledges midwives as being an oppressed group, which can lead to ‘horizontal violence’ and fear of change. Horizontal violence is where an oppressed group do not have the power to change their situation and so monitor and criticise each other, rather than those oppressing them.

Current midwifery culture

Kirkham (1999), in her ethnographic study, interviewed 168 midwives from diverse areas to seek their understanding of the midwifery culture in the NHS in England. This data was analysed using a grounded theory approach. She found ten categories. The first category she discusses is 'service and sacrifice', which is where midwives continue to offer care and commitment, irrespective of personal sacrifice. This can be seen in other studies as well (Hildingsson and Häggström 1999, Bolton 2000, John and Parsons 2006).

Midwives' perception was that they needed to be selfless and self-sacrificing, and not to seek support. Alongside this, experienced midwives felt that, when colleagues said they were being supportive, they interpreted it as monitoring and policing. This leads to great pressure to conform to behavioural norms. In this culture, where there is pressure to conform, the midwives achieved doing 'good' by stealth. This doing 'good' by stealth was a strategy that midwives used with obstetricians to protect women, but it would appear that they were now having to use it with their supervisors too (Kirkham 1999). This has also been seen in other studies (Hunter 2004).

Midwives were seen to be experiencing an overwhelming sense of helplessness, and the market, management and culture of midwifery reinforced this sense of oppression. The culture of midwifery is one where the traditional values of midwives to support and care continue, but in an organisation that has very different values. The midwives' role is to facilitate confidence and increase the ability of the women they care for, but loyalty to their organisational culture prevents them from seeking, or seeing themselves as deserving of, this support and care (Kirkham 1999).

The oppressive culture in midwifery, clearly outlined by Kirkham in her study, can be found in most of the literature pertaining to research into women-centred care in midwifery. It may, though, be too simplistic to identify this oppression as caused by one factor, as suggested in Kirkham's study: the NHS management. Throughout the development of professional midwifery there have been many influential factors affecting the professional culture, including midwives from different socio-economic groups (Hunter and Leap 1993), inter-professional rivalry (Rhodes 1995, Tew 1998), political agendas (DoH 2004) and what women want, which is again influenced by their cultural expectations (Hochschild 2003).

Despite the current political climate encouraging midwives to be women-centred and to encourage 'normal birth', choice, control and breast feeding (DoH 2003, 2006, ICM 2006), there is still the expectation that this will occur within a goal-orientated, audit-driven and litigious social climate (Kirkham 2000). Kirkham (2009) does offer a way forward, based on midwifery research and reflecting on the authors' writing in Hunter and Deery's book 'Emotions in midwifery and reproduction' (2009). She states there is the need for political changes to allow trusting, ongoing relationships and autonomy of practice through decentralisation and reduction of high-tech solutions. Kirkham (2009) also highlights changes that midwives need to undertake. They need to reduce defensive habits and learn creative, emotional responses through skilled facilitation and excellent role- models.

With the dual ideologies in midwifery, sitting within the already discussed cultural hegemony, which are confounded by the wealth of governmental guidance, it is not surprising that midwives are unclear whether they should offer the emotional care they perceive as being necessary.

Clear boundary between professional (midwife) and client (woman)

Midwives attempting to offer emotional support within the current culture of midwifery services in the NHS, can be seen to be struggling with being both 'with woman' and 'with institution'. The midwives in Hildingsson and Häggström's study (1999) did not seem to go through this struggle. They identified that midwives in their study were taking on a 'good mother' role with the women to whom they were offering care, but Hunter (2006) suggests this is also problematic in the current healthcare climate in the UK. Hunter (2004) explains that midwives are expected to work in partnership with women, rather than to 'mother' them. The midwife-woman relationship was more fully explored in chapter 3. Swedish maternity services may not have the same ideological underpinning as midwives in the UK, but the ICM clearly guides midwives to work in a 'with woman' way, therefore there may be differing cultural perceptions of what a 'good mother' is.

The midwives in my study appeared to believe they needed to be both professional and knowledgeable, and 'with woman' and caring. They sought a relationship of partnership (Fleming 1998b) and to come alongside women (Fleming 1998a). Bolton (2000) recognised this need to balance being a professional within an organisation and its expectations, at the same time as offering human caring or 'with women' care. She identified that, whilst the (gynaecological) nurses in her study offered a "gift", an extra element of care, it did not receive status and was not required by the organisation, but they felt it was necessary. Unlike the midwives in my study they did not struggle with this; they did not concern themselves with whether offering this care would reduce their professionalism. Indeed, they said that they did not believe anyone could be a nurse unless they were prepared to offer this extra care from within themselves. It might, therefore, appear that this struggle with ideologies is specific to the midwifery profession in the UK, rather than the task undertaken, as the tasks these nurses were undertaking were similar to some conducted by midwives.

The midwives in my study seem drawn to using their personal experiences, feelings and intuition as women, to come alongside other women and support them, but they were concerned whether this would be in conflict with what they believed their profession expected of them. For some, this led to a cautious approach to caring which can be seen through the explanation of one of the midwives that she recognised some of the restrictions placed on her, due to professional boundaries, but she also recognised that there was a need to work within a structure. She said,

> "When you start putting boundaries and restrictions in you create problems… yet you know you work within a structure that is set up but you have to."

A couple of the midwives in my study, did seem to be taking on the role of the 'good mother' and experienced the problem of where the boundary was between being 'professional' and being 'with woman'. Whilst they desired to encourage and support the women to achieve independence, there remained the desire to offer care. Making the decision of when to stand back, and when to intervene, was difficult and created a struggle for them. This becomes particularly apparent in one midwife's desire to help and practically assist the woman she was caring for, conflicting with the recognition that she must facilitate independence. Diane shared her thoughts that

> "In a way I was perhaps anxious because I always worry when you've got to manually get a baby on and every bodies struggling with this sort of thing, did I do the right thing there" and "I felt I was wrong there perhaps I should have let her really try a bit more herself."

Hildingsson and Häggström (1999) also identified that playing the role of 'good mother' had some negative consequences, such as midwives admonishing the women. This can also be seen to some degree in this study, where a midwife described, when attempting to balance helping and facilitating independence, how the woman became fearful of 'being told off', which may indicate that she appeared to the woman as a critical mother- figure.

Whether these midwives are considered to be working in a motherly, 'good mother', manner or not, in them can be seen some of the struggle midwives have with attempting to maintain professionalism, whilst simultaneously coming alongside the women and offering emotionally supportive care. This struggle with boundaries can sometimes find midwives on one side of it or the other. Sometimes midwives will put on one side their 'institutional' ideology and at other times will put on one side their 'with woman' ideology, as can be seen when they are toeing the organisational line.

Toeing the organisational line

Carol needed to put effort into emotion work due to others, apparently colleagues, upsetting the woman she was caring for. She said,

> "Different people were coming in; one would say this, one would say that and so she had a lot of upset about that. And then um I think one person in particular upset her"

This demonstrates that it is not just the midwife-woman relationship that creates emotion work for midwives, as identified by Hunter (2004); it can also be colleagues. Carol, in her description of her care, appeared to go on, as with another midwife, to use rationalisation to cope with the situation. She offers a rational explanation of what happened and why she responded to the woman in the way she did.

Carol appeared to desire to support and defend her colleagues, whilst at the same time advocating for and supporting the woman for whom she was caring. This led Carol to rationalise the woman's experience by saying her colleagues were unable to make the experience different and the woman lacked the ability to manage the situation. Carol then went on to defend the woman by suggesting that other women might have the same inability and the woman probably had 'underlying issues', which also offered a reason for this inability. Carol may have felt it unprofessional to say to the woman that her colleagues should have been more consistent in her care. This is despite governmental and professional body guidelines stating that maternity care should be woman- focused. In this example, Carol can be seen to be 'toeing the organisational line', or behaving in a 'with institution' or 'with profession' way.

There were other examples in my study where conflicting ideologies created extra emotion work for the midwife. A number of the midwives experienced dissonance, due to their desire to follow the 'with woman' ideology and the need to also follow the 'with institution' ideology (Hunter 2005). For them there was the need to draw on 'feeling rules', which can be contradictory if opposing ideologies are held. This can cause increased emotion work and stress and may lead to burn out. Managing the differing ideologies identified by Hunter (2005) can be seen as being problematic for the midwives.

In Emily's situation she needed to provide emotion work due to the organisational structure not being what the woman had hoped for. Emily said,

> "She felt that the midwife she had met first off, although we got on very well, she felt that, I have gone through my history with this one midwife and now have to again. She got herself in a terrible state about it".

For Betty, she did not encourage the woman she was caring for to breast feed, despite the woman appearing to want to do this and Betty believing it would not be a problem. This was because the paediatrician had told the woman not to breast-feed and Betty felt she should not contradict this. Likewise, Hetty had to take a role she was uncomfortable with, due to professional expectations.

The midwives did not explicitly acknowledge the differing ideologies in midwifery, but these can clearly be seen in their descriptions of their care. Despite the extra emotion work and the personal dissonance created between being 'with institution' and 'with woman', they still appeared to desire to provide emotional support to the women. It can be seen, though, in my study, that it may have affected the care given by the midwives.

Within the culture of midwifery services, with its dual ideology and the perceived need to offer a reason for giving emotional support, I found a number of other areas in which the midwives struggled.

Differing perceptions between women and midwives

An experience for some of the midwives in this study, which caused them some concern or stress, was the lack of understanding between themselves and the women of each other's worldviews. Examples include that Carol could not empathise with the woman's view that her birth was traumatic and that Emily could not understand why the woman she had met was distressed about their interaction.

These examples offer a demonstration that, at times, midwives struggled to understand the women's perceptions and frequently the women were unable to understand what the midwives were trying to communicate to them. Interestingly McCourt (2005), in her study which focused on interviewing and observing midwives, recognised that it was the evaluation of these interactions that led the midwives to believe the meeting had gone well or otherwise. She said that a good visit equated with a 'good' client who was "relaxed and confident, who asked the appropriate questions tended to put the midwife at her ease too" (McCourt 2005: 1316). It may be that, due to Emily gaining articulate, relaxed and confident responses from the woman, she believed the appointment had gone well, whereas the woman had left unhappy.

This lack of mutual understanding has been found in other studies. Fleming (1998b) and Kirkham et al (2002b) also found, when interviewing women and their midwives about their experiences of midwifery care, that there were a number of contradictions. The midwives and women had different expectations and reflections on their experiences. This desire or perceived necessity, for the women to understand the midwives' perspective and the need for midwives to understand the women's experiences, created extra effort and emotion work for midwives.

This struggle can also be seen when the midwives were giving emotional support to women. The midwives felt the women had unrealistic expectation of both themselves and midwifery care. The midwives thought the unrealistic expectations the women had of themselves, their stereotype of a mother and of a midwife may lead them to experience emotional distress or mental health problems.

Mother stereotype

Motherhood is enacted within a social and political arena, which influences the dominant discourses on mothering (Littlewood and McHugh 1997, Magill-Cuerden 2006, Miller 2007). With monumental changes occurring for the women (Barclay et al.1996, Bondas and Eriksson 2001, Cronin 2003, Miller 2007) and cultural pressures influenced by the discourses of medicine and nature (Miller 2007), women strive to be 'good mothers' (Brown et al 1997, Bondas and Eriksson 2001, Marchant 2004, Magill-Cuerden 2006, Miller 2007). This 'good mother' appears to be an unachievable stereotype.

The stereotype of the 'good mother', along with the medicine and nature discourses of becoming a mother, as described in chapter one, can be recognised in the descriptions of the midwives in my study. They acknowledged the stereotype and attempted to gain more realistic expectations in the women they were caring for. It can be seen that they also believed that women having too high expectations of themselves leads to emotional distress and perhaps postnatal depression.

Despite the assumption that unrealistic expectations of self and other leads to emotional distress and postnatal depression, this is not supported by Brown et al (1997). They found that most women, regardless of whether they had depressive symptoms or not, held the same idealistic stereotype of a mother. It may be that there is another underlying cause for women to become depressed around the time of having a baby, but the midwives in my study appeared to accept this 'given' knowledge or assumption. This may have caused them to try to address the issue of unrealistic expectations to reduce emotional distress, whereas they could, more effectively, be addressing another issue.

Midwife Stereotype

The unrealistic expectations with which the midwives in my study appeared to struggle, included the stereotypes about midwives and midwifery practice. The midwives gave accounts of where the women had unrealistic expectations of them. These expectations were quite varied, but most related to expectations that the midwives could not fulfil (working across boundaries, continuous attendance, knowledge about anything related to pregnancy). However, one description identified the lack of care the woman expected; she did not expect the level of care that was offered to her.

The midwives also identified that women have certain expectations about their personalities; they have a stereotype of midwives. Each of the midwives who mentioned this said they did not fulfil the stereotypical personality of a professional midwife. Emily said,

> "A lot of women say they expect a midwife to be very posh and umm very umm prissy,"

which she did not believe herself to be, whereas Hetty said that she believed women expected them to be focused on the baby and physical health issues.

Antenatal classes

Antenatal, or parentcraft classes, were an area within which the midwives expressed their frustration at not being able to gain a shared worldview with the women. They felt unable to adequately prepare women for the journey to motherhood mentally and emotionally. Carol explained that, despite offering information about pain and other issues at classes the woman, was still shocked. Carol felt that, despite her explanations, the woman still developed expectations of herself that she was unable to fulfil and this created the need for emotional support later. Likewise, Emily said that the woman she was working with had expectations of how things would be after the baby arrived and, despite her attempts to ease the woman into understanding in antenatal classes, she was still unhappy and needed extra support. Fiona appeared to sum the situation up when she stated that each experience is too different to be adequately prepared for through group antenatal classes. Although Betty was not talking about antenatal classes, she also found problems with information-giving and understanding, which meant that she had to take much longer explaining and identified a higher need for emotional care.

The lack of understanding of each other's world views also compounded another area in which the midwives struggled. Time was limited and the midwives explained how offering emotional support was time-consuming. This struggle with differing worldviews can be seen to increase the time needed and the midwives emotion work when providing emotional support.

Use of personal rules or instincts

The midwives in my study did not appear to have a clear understanding of how to manage their emotional support, despite the prolific amount of policies and government guidance available on midwifery care. This appeared to be the situation, as the midwives described personal rules or instincts guiding them to manage their relationships, instead of describing guidance or knowledge.

To deal with the dilemma or struggle between being 'with woman' or 'being professional', the midwives developed personal rules for themselves, such as Emily who said she used self-disclosure to aid the relationship, but she avoided talking about her own pregnancy. Hetty recognised that the relationship she had with the woman was not what was expected, but that she used her gut instinct to guide her. Likewise Gina accessed her instincts to guide her; she also identified that the woman was driven by her instincts as well.

Becoming a mother is widely acknowledged as an emotional time and those supporting women at this time may not only experience the women's emotions, but personal emotions as well.

Sharing of emotional moments

The women and midwives in my study appeared to experience a range of emotions from guilt, fear and distress to being peaceful, happy and cheerful. Although the midwives were attempting to facilitate comfort and positive emotions in the women, this did not always occur. Indeed, one midwife appeared to have induced fear. Diane explained,

> "And she said to me I hope you are not going to tell me off" and "she was also feeling a bit guilty because she thought I was going to tell her off".

Hildingsson and Häggström (1999) also identified midwives in this position. They found that, when the midwives in their study took on the role of 'good mother' they sometimes admonished the women in their care. It may be that the woman Diane was working with saw her as a critical mother- figure rather than a partner in her care. This situation can be seen to have occurred for Diane as she was attempting to promote independence in the woman, by providing her with information about breast-feeding, as guided by both the Nice guidelines (2006) and her professional bodies (RCM, ICM 2006).

Diane can be seen to be struggling not only with the emotions generated, fear and anxiety, but also with how to resolve the problems for the woman. She is obviously, from the woman's perspective and her own words, attempting to act in accordance with two competing groups of rules which come from the differing ideologies in midwifery. Organisationally and personally she feels she should be promoting total breast-feeding of the baby, but at the same time she is attempting to behave within the ideology of 'with woman', as discussed by Hunter (2004). As one woman with another, she appears to desire to achieve comfort for the woman and reduce her distress.

This dissonance between conflicting ideologies can be seen to be creating emotional conflict and work for Diane. She appears to desire to tell the woman she should give herself more time, to carry on trying to fully breast-feed, as this will be more fulfilling for her and the baby. Diane, though, recognises the anxiety in the woman and compromises her own feelings and the organisation's standpoint, to address the feelings of the woman. Diane then uses a common coping strategy, as described by Mann (2004), of rationalisation to reduce her own and the woman's dissonance, as the woman, as well as feeling fearful of Diane, was also feeling guilty. Diane achieved this rationalisation by saying that, as the mother, the woman knew what was best for her baby.

As can be seen through Diane's interactions, holding opposing ideologies without the recognition of this by policy makers, managers and educationalists, can lead to limited support and guidance and problems in care-giving. Another example of the midwives working with the feelings of the women they were caring for is demonstrated by Betty. Betty said,

> "Luckily they never felt they needed to apologise to me so hopefully that means, that was because they didn't feel that I was being short with them or losing my patience. Because they kept thanking me all the time, 'thank you for doing this' and 'thank you for doing that' and all the time they were really thankful and very grateful so hopefully, you know, that was the support that I gave but hopefully that I didn't make them feel, you know, that they were being a nuisance".

Betty clearly described the couple as being very grateful for her help; she believed this demonstrated she was doing a good job, but it did create emotion work for her. An indication of this can be found in Betty's comment that she hoped she did not make them feel they were being a nuisance. This obviously was not a balanced relationship, which is advocated by Hunter (2006). Betty appeared to have to put a lot of effort into all the care given to this couple, including emotional support. Betty, herself, acknowledged it took extra time and effort to communicate with them. She did, though, appear at times to be using ‘feeling rules’, as she was acting in a manner she felt she needed to (Hochschild 2003, Savage 2004). Betty does not say she felt ‘short’ or at risk of being ‘impatient’ with them, but she does indicate she is concerned that they may feel she is. She assesses whether they feel she is impatient by their need to apologise, which they do not do. It could be, though, that their need to constantly express gratitude is demonstrating this. This obviously caused emotion work for Betty, as she tried to facilitate a feeling of being valued and worthy in the couple, at the same time as having to put in a lot of effort to provide the care they appeared to need. Betty said,

> “I didn’t find the experience of looking after her in any way traumatic, in fact quite the opposite; I found it quite enhancing really because they were such a delightful couple and because she was, both of them were very receptive”.

Betty clearly identified that the emotional responses of the woman indicated to her that she was providing emotional support and that she had gained a rapport with her.

Good rapport leads to positive outcomes

My study offers a detailed account of the midwives’ experiences. The context or culture within which they occur has been discussed earlier in this chapter. The detail of how midwives give emotional support or care to women becoming mothers was discussed in chapter four. Experience of providing emotional support to women becoming mothers can be seen to be exhausting and time-consuming, but can bring pleasure to both. It involves emotion work for the midwives but when a good rapport develops it facilitates comfort in the women and a sense of satisfaction for the midwives. This appears to relate to what Hunter (2006) calls a balanced reciprocal relationship. Fleming (1998a) and Pairman (2000) also recognise the desirability of reciprocity within the midwife-woman relationship.

A reciprocal relationship is one in which the midwife needs to do least emotion work and is therefore most emotionally healthy for midwife and woman (Fleming 1998a, Pairman 2000, Hunter 2006). The midwives in my study did not appear to have totally reciprocal relationships, but this may be due to them identifying times where they needed to offer emotional support. However, they did conclude their description with the indication that they achieved a more reciprocal relationship by the end of their care.

When the women and midwives gained a good rapport or balanced reciprocal relationship (Hunter 2006), both achieved positive emotional outcomes (Fleming 1998a, Pairman 2000) and this led to a greater desire in the midwife to care for the woman. Despite the relationship between the midwives and the woman not being truly balanced, especially initially, they did eventually appear to become more reciprocal relationships.

Emotion to evaluate care

The midwives in my study appeared to use the responses of the women extensively to evaluate their care. When the woman seemed happy, the midwives assessed themselves to have done a good job. Gina felt she had done a good job because the mother was happy as indicated by this statement,

> "I asked her how she felt about things so that she could express whatever she was feeling um she was just happy about things then".

Diane also said,

> "But then I did feel satisfied I left her feeling happy with the decisions she had made, she felt that she had made the right decision really".

Emotion work

Theories associated with emotion work will be considered in chapter six, so have not been discussed here, but this chapter has recognised that there are many elements of the midwives' role that create emotion work for them. As already established, emotion work can be experienced in response to 'feeling rules' associated with care for women and 'feeling rules' associated with colleagues' expectations (Hunter 2004).

The midwives in this study dealt with many struggles and expended emotion work effort in their desire to offer emotionally supportive care. In doing this, the most influential struggle appeared to be the struggle between what they believed their profession expected of them and their desire to come alongside women. They appeared to believe that their profession expected them to 'toe' the organisation's 'line', not to undermine colleagues (whether midwives or doctors), and to see a large number of women with a professional distance, a clear boundary between professional and client.

Summary

The midwives in my study appear to have a number of significant factors, influencing their experience of giving emotional support to women becoming mothers. The culture within which this care occurs has an impact on all those associated with it. The methodology I used, descriptive phenomenology, also guides the researcher to identify the context or culture within which the study is being undertaken.

It can be seen that the culture has a long history, but has probably seen the most significant changes over the last century which influences all aspects of the midwives' care. The decision of whether to offer emotional support, how and where, are all set within the midwifery culture with its underpinning philosophy, along with framing and feeling rules.

Their professional culture is influenced and guided by research, particularly that which underpins policy. An example is the need for control, choice and continuity in Changing Childbirth (DoH 1993). The NICE guidelines and NSF lead midwives to ensure care is provided, particularly to needy groups of women, in a flexible manner. The midwives were strongly guided by institutional rules, whether explicitly or implicitly laid down. As all the midwives appeared to be following the same guidance, there appears to be some sort of unstated 'framing rules' accepted.

Despite this, they are also led by the women's expressed emotions, intuition and personal rules to come alongside women. Through this apparent need to follow policy and institutional expectation, as well as to follow their intuition, midwives find they experience the need to provide emotion work, as well as therapeutic emotional labour. Nurses working in similar situations appear to come together and state that their professional expectation of each other is to offer the 'gift' of emotion work, recognising it takes time and effort which, in turn, reduces some of the emotional labour (Bolton 2000).

Although midwives' experience of providing emotional support is that it takes extra time and effort, it is not totally unrewarded. Despite literature suggesting the work is unrecognised and under-valued (Bolton 2000, John and Parsons 2006), the midwives appeared to gain a reward from the women's expressions of pleasure, comfort and rapport gained and not from the institution for whom they work.

In my study the experiences of giving emotional support to women becoming mothers are different from those of the midwives in Hildingsson and Häggström's (1999) study, probably due to cultural differences, but how they summed it up would be similar. To offer this type of care, was summed up by the statement, "to be a 'good mother' demands an involvement that can be both emotionally exhausting and time-consuming but also joyful" (Hildingsson and Häggström (1999: 88).

CHAPTER SIX

WHAT IS EMOTION WORK?

Introduction

When considering emotional care it is important to recognise, not only what it looks like when it is provided, but also how that care is achieved by the care-giver and the impact it might have on them. This has had various labels over the last couple of decades, with researchers such as Hochschild (1979) and Pam Smith (1992) describing emotional labour in the work place (aeroplanes and hospitals). Others more recently labelled working with emotions in maternity care as emotion work, such as Hunter (2001). Regardless of the label, it is important that the carer's efforts are recognised and appreciated to enhance the well-being of both care-giver and recipient (Hochschild 1983).

Theories of emotion

Charles Darwin, accepted as the founder of evolutionary theory, was one of the earliest researchers to explicitly explore emotions and, due to the cross-cultural nature of his findings, decided that emotional expression was inherited (Savage 2004). Along with Darwin, the psychodynamic approach of Freud and, to some extent, the biopsychological approach of James and Lange (Carlson et al 2004), offer an instinctual understanding of emotions (Hochschild 1979), whereas behavioural and cognitive approaches, whilst accepting the availability of the biological apparatus, would recognise emotions as learnt responses to situations or experiences. The social psychological theories of the person, including behavioural and cognitive approaches, can be considered interactional models of emotion.

As can be seen by the number of differing theoretical approaches, psychologists have difficulty in finding a consensual understanding of the concept of emotion (Carlson et al 2004). For psychologists, there would appear to be the perennial debate between nature and nurture for emotions, as with other psychological theories of the person. The most recent theorists, though, would appear to promote an interactional approach to understanding emotions, which suggest that elements of the person's internal make up, and the environment in which they live, influence their emotional experience and expression.

According to Strongman (1996) culture would appear to be an underlying linking factor in most theoretical work in the development of understanding of emotions. Within the available theories there is, though, the need to acknowledge that these are personal and psychophysiological experiences. This would appear to suggest that cultural theories overlap both nature and nurture approaches highlighted by psychologists. Philosophical, historical, anthropological and sociological disciplines all offer a cultural theory of emotions (Strongman 1996). "Culture is socially determined and shapes many aspects of our identity, including our beliefs, values and behaviour. It encompasses many factors, including race, ethnicity, religion, gender, sexuality, age, generation, class, life experience and lifestyle" (Thurgood 2009:630).

Social or Sociological theorists suggest that, despite the psycho-physiological experience of emotion, these are not reducible, they should not be reviewed outside of their social context and that social process should be considered as well. They have developed theories considering social processes, such as power and status (Kemper 1978), social cohesion (Goffman 1970), social control (Scheff 1990), symbolic interaction (Rosenberg 1990) and culture (Hochschild 1983). Historical, anthropological, psychological and sociological disciplines all allow for a phenomenological exploration of emotions, which is the underpinning approach accepted within this book.

Historical studies also suggest that emotional cultures have gender differentials (Strongman 1996, Trew and Kremer 1998), so any theory of emotions should include personal (psychophysiological) and sociocultural (gender etc) elements.

Gross (2001) writes from a psychological perspective, that emotions involve a subjective experience, physiological changes and an associated behavioural change and different emotional theories are due to the differing emphasis put on each component. Social and cultural influences can be seen to be enacted through Gross's (2001) label of subjective experience. The writing of Hochschild (1979:551), a sociologist, is seminal in the area of emotion work or management and she defines emotion as “bodily co-operation with an image, a thought, a memory – a co-operation of which the individual is aware”. These two definitions do not seem mutually exclusive and can be accepted as useful definitions for this exploration. The working definition accepted here is, therefore, that emotion is the interaction between physiological changes (internal and / or external) in response to an experience (mentally and/ or physically).

Emotion management

Hochschild (1983) explored the psychological theories of the person to develop her sociological understanding of emotions. She also considered how psychological theory could enhance her understanding of how a person might manage their emotions. This management of emotions can be seen as twofold; in providing emotional care there is the management of personal emotions as well the management of the emotions of the person being cared for. Hochschild’s understanding was particularly influenced by the dramaturgical theory of Goffman (a social psychological theory), to some extent the neo-Freudians (psychodynamic approach) and Lazarus’s interactional model (Hochschild 1979). Hochschild’s research has focused mainly on what she labelled emotional labour or emotion management and the commercialisation of this effort. Her research provides a contemporary and extended viewpoint for Goffman’s theory of ‘playing roles’, whilst accepting some elements of psychodynamic and interactional theory. Therefore, despite being a sociological theorist she has been greatly influenced by psychological theory.

Goffman (1959), a behavioural psychologist, suggested that people were always ‘playing’ a part or role and the person could only be defined by the role they were playing at the time. At different times people are ‘acting’ or ‘playing’ different parts and could, therefore, be defined socially as a different person. He developed the concept of ‘The Art of Impression Management’ (Goffman 1959) which has, as would be expected, similarities with Hochschild’s emotion management. There is, though, a significant difference between their views of the person. Hochschild acknowledges the person as having a distinct personal emotional world, whereas Goffman only acknowledges the person as the role they are playing. Goffman (1959) writes of the rules of acting a role, which could be described as ‘surface acting’ using Hochschild’s terms, whereas she describes ‘surface acting’ and ‘deep acting’ in her writing. This is an important issue when we consider the role fulfilled when emotionally supporting women and the impact this might have on them. It has been highlighted by Hunter (2006) and Sandall (1997) that high levels of emotion work or 'deep acting' can lead to 'burn- out' and ill- health in the care- provider, including midwives.

Whilst Goffman provided a basis for Hochschild's cultural theory of emotions, others, such as Freud, Darwin and Lazarus, were also influential. Darwin believed that emotions were universal gestures that led to a behaviour or action. For example, the emotion of love, with its associated gestures, leads to copulation. Whereas Freud, although his theory did evolve over his lifetime, was concerned with the meaning of emotions and implied emotions are signals. The experience of an emotion for Freud signalled an inner or external state, for example if the emotion of anxiety was experienced, the person might interpret this signal as a sign of impending danger (Hochschild 1983). Whether Darwin's theory of emotions as motivating or Freud's theory of emotions as signals, are accepted, the definition already stated for emotion is not diminished. "Emotion is the interaction between physiological changes (internal and / or external) in response to an experience (mentally and/ or physically)". Both Darwin and Freud are explaining the role emotions play.

Lazarus's model of emotional experiencing is an interactional model, as it takes into consideration not only the environment and internal physiological responses, but also learnt coping strategies (Lazarus 1966). Hochschild (1983) drew on all these theorists and others to develop her cultural theory and research of emotions and how these are managed. Goffman, Freud, Lazarus and Hochschild could all offer insights into the emotional experiences of emotionally supporting motherhood. If Goffman's approach is applied to offering emotionally supportive care, we might interpret the care-giver as playing a role or part with no empathetic or personal emotional experience. Care-givers could be seen to be following the social or learnt rules for the role that they are undertaking.

A Freudian or psychodynamic view of the care-giver's emotional behaviour such as compassion, which could be demonstrated when offering emotionally supportive care, might be that it is a signal. This signal could be viewed as a demonstration of the carer's need for kindness, calm and compassion. It could also be viewed as a signal as recognition of need in the woman and an outward sign of the care-giver's internalised identification with their own mother.

Hochschild's (1983) understanding of emotions led to her development of a cultural theory of emotional labour or emotion management. This has been influential in the development of understanding of emotional labour, or emotion management, in all areas of western society.

Emotion Work

The cultural theory of emotional labour or emotion management, by Hochschild (1983), has been influential in the development of understanding of emotional labour or emotion management in all areas of western society. She does not distinguish between emotional labour and emotion management and uses the terms interchangeably, but she usually uses the term emotional labour to label her theory. She does, though, differentiate between emotional labour and emotion work, defining emotional labour as emotion management in the public arena and governed by display and feeling rules. Emotion work is what is undertaken in the private arena.

Hochschild's (1979) theory of emotional labour offers categories from which to understand emotions. She suggests that emotional behaviour, as with other cultural behaviour, follows certain rules. Hochschild (1979) describes what she labels 'display' rules and 'feeling' rules. Display rules are similar to the social rules identified by Goffman (1959) and have been categorised as 'superficial acting'. These are the rules for the explicit behaviour that a culture or organisation requires of a person in a given situation. Feeling rules can be recognised as 'superficial acting' or 'deep acting' and these inform the person about how they should feel. Superficial acting is where the person outwardly behaves as if they hold a certain feeling, but do not feel it inside, whereas deep acting is where the person adapts their inner feelings to that which is expected. Hochschild (1983) indicates that, in the current culture, more organisations are setting feeling rules for their employees alongside display rules. She also highlights that if a person performs the feeling rules of an organisation by deep acting, they may be at risk of losing their 'self', or personal integrity.

Feeling rules underpin ideologies and can be considered as part of an interpretative framework. An interpretative framework can be explained in terms of 'framing rules' and 'feeling rules' (Hochschild 1979). Display rules offer guidance on how to behave, but are not a focus within this interpretative framework. Framing rules are general rules, which offer definition and meaning to a situation, whereas feeling rules offer an understanding of what might be an appropriate way to feel in a given situation. For example, an interpretative framework for a midwife might be where the framing rules define a situation as one in which she has responsibility for the woman and provide the meaning that a woman is distressed. Feeling rules may tell the midwife that she should feel caring and compassionate towards the woman. This may lead to the midwife using emotional labour, or management, if this is not how she feels.

Framing and feeling rules are, according to Hochschild (1983), used extensively in social situations, but she was particularly interested in the commercialisation of these rules and the effort involved in emotional labour. She found that employers who were buying the emotional labour of their employees expect not only a certain type of behaviour in their staff, but also that their staff are sincere and feel the dictated emotion.

This can be seen in therapeutic relationships in health care. The counselling theories of Rogers (1951) and Egan (1977) both expect the counsellor to offer non-judgmental, positive regard for the client, regardless of what the client may have done. This has to be offered congruently; with sincerity. The counsellor in a counselling situation (framing rule), therefore, has to feel positive regard for the client (feeling rule). Although Rogers and Egan were not using Hochschild's interpretative framework, their theoretical stance can be interpreted using it. Hochschild's theory has, though, been applied to healthcare, including midwifery, by a number of authors but most significantly by Hunter (2001, 2004, 2005, 2006) who will be considered later in this chapter.

Health Care Professionals work with emotions

Researchers and writers in health care have built on Hochschild's foundational sociological work. There has been a lack of distinction amongst these authors over the definition of the terms emotional labour, emotion work and emotion management (Mann 2004, 2005, Hunter and Deery 2009). Despite this lack of clarity over definition, there appears to be agreement that, whilst emotional labour is essential, it creates a great deal of work stress for the provider (Smith 1992, Mann 2004, 2005, Hunter 2006). To explore this area of health professionals' effort in more detail, it would be helpful to initially consider the earliest literature available first.

Nursing seems to provide the earliest consideration of this area in health care. One of the earliest nurses to explore this area was Pam Smith, in

1992; she examined the literature on emotional labour. This was undertaken to establish whether it was the same as what is labelled "nursing care", which is regarded as essential for patient well-being. Smith was considered to be an influential leader in the development of understanding of emotional labour in health care, so much so, that she was invited to write the preface for the ground-breaking midwifery book by Hunter and Deery in 2009. Smith (1992) concluded that nursing care and emotional labour are essentially the same experiences in different situations. She also said that giving emotional labour was, at times, at great cost.

More recently, a study was undertaken to explore the area of work with emotions undertaken by nurses (Bolton 2000). The nurses in this study had some overlap in their workload to midwives, in that they mostly cared for women who had miscarriages and fertility issues (ICM 2006). Nurses appeared to offer emotion work as a 'gift' to those for whom they care, a term also used by Hochschild (2003). Gynaecological nurses, with a variety of grades and experiences, were interviewed and observed. Ideologically, nursing is seen as feminine (framing rule) with the associated qualities of being caring, loving and kind (feeling rules) (Bolton 2000). It is seen as a vocation (framing) which raises a number of expectations of nurses, by those being cared for and the nurses of themselves. Nurses believe they should always be kind and caring but also calm and detached (feeling rules) (Bolton 2000). These are the feeling rules (Hochschild 1979) for this nursing group. One quote from a ward sister which demonstrates this underpinning ideology of nurses was "the essential basis of nursing is caring. You can't be a nurse if you don't care" (Bolton 2000:583). This untaught but professionally acknowledged expectation is suggested to be necessary but may invoke, as already identified (Hochschild 1979, 1983, 2003, Mann 2004, 2005, Hunter 2004, 2006), what has been labelled as emotional labour or emotion work.

The nurses in this study were undertaking what Hochschild would label emotional labour, but they were seen to be doing more than managing their emotions. They were offering something extra that was labelled a 'gift'. Nurses were undertaking emotion work as well as emotion management or emotional labour, to use Hochschild's definitions. The nurses offered their 'gift' of emotion work to each other in a reciprocal manner, but they offered it to patients and their families with little or no expectation of reciprocity, hence the term 'gift' (Bolton 2000). Hochschild (2003) identified similar situations, where usually gifts are reciprocal, but sometimes the gift is given without expectation of reward, when she was exploring emotions in the private arena, which she labelled emotion work.

As already highlighted, nursing care and emotional labour can be considered synonymous (Smith 1992). Most of the nurses in Bolton's study recognised that caring for patients brought them anxiety but also brought the greatest potential for job satisfaction. Hochschild (2003) wrote, "the sharing of gifts is a cultural phenomenon but offering a gift is sign of love. The sense of genuine giving and receiving is a part of love. So it is through the idea of a gift that we use culture to express love" (Hochschild 2003:104). There are a number of writers who accept that care is a moderated type of love (Campbell 1984, Freshwater and Stickley 2004).

Care, particularly emotional care, can be seen as a type of loving interaction which appears to be an important part of nursing and midwifery practice. It can be dangerous for caring professions, such as nursing, to focus too much on professionalism and technological skills (Bolton 2000) and some nurses defend their professionalism, but celebrate their ability to 'care too much' (Bolton 2000).

This dichotomy of professional technical care and emotional care, in the form of a gift, can create emotion work for nurses and midwives, particularly those who come alongside women becoming mothers (Hunter 2004). These competing approaches or ideologies can be explained in the terms identified by Hochschild (1979). Hochschild (1979), as already stated, recognised that feeling rules and framing rules underpin ideology. If a care-giver supporting a woman becoming a mother was experiencing an ideological dissonance, they might have had competing framing and feeling rules. The nurses in Bolton's study appeared aware of this dissonance and chose their set of feeling rules and, therefore, their ideological stance.

Emotion work in midwives

A review of the knowledge of midwives' emotion work, those most likely to be needed to provide emotional care to women on their journey to motherhood, was conducted by Billie Hunter in 2001. She chose to use the term emotion work as she saw midwives as undertaking their role in both public (hospitals) and private (personal homes) places. Despite the quality of the childbirth experience and the relationship between the mother and midwife being crucial for the mother's well-being, she found that emotion work was under-represented in the research.

Hunter (2001) stated there is a high level of emotion work for midwives and this continues to increase with the changes that are occurring in the maternity services, with the focus on holistic care, caseload management and the need for continuity. She understood emotion work, or emotional labour, to be anything that has an impact on the midwives' emotional state, but she does not offer a definition of emotion. Hunter was more concerned with the midwives' perception of their emotional state and appears accepting of their interpretation of this.

There is a need to develop midwives' understanding of emotion in the workplace for the well-being, not only of the mothers, but also of themselves (Hunter 2001, Deery 2009, Kirkham 2009). The expectation is that this increased understanding will improve the midwives' working lives and allow them to meet the needs of the women and families with whom they work. This is crucial, as a negative experience during this time for the mother, whether during pregnancy, birth or post birth, may lead to emotional distress (Barclay et al 1996, 1997, Shields et al 1997).

Hunter has conducted a number of studies in the area of emotion work since 2001 and has had a number of related papers published. In 2004, she presented a paper entitled "The Conflicting Ideologies in Midwifery as a Source of Emotion Work for Midwives". In this paper, Hunter's (2004) findings are interesting in that the expectation is that emotion work has its source within the relationships between client and professional, whereas she found the emotion work was primarily due to co-existing conflicting ideologies. As has been previously established, differing ideologies suggest differing framing and feeling rules should be applied. This could be seen as a potential situation for unhealthy cognitive and emotional dissonance.

In 2005, Hunter went on to explore the area of conflicting ideologies further and, through her studies, she identified that relationships between midwifery colleagues were of key importance. These relationships can clearly be seen, particularly in hospital-based care, where hierarchical relationships enforce a convergence of ideologies, to produce dissonance in the more junior midwives. Senior midwives were found to use unwritten rules and sanctions to maintain their senior positions (Hunter

2005), which may be considered to be similar to the strategies undertaken by those providing flight-attendance training in Hochschild's (1983, 2003) early study. They underpinned these strategies by referring to their greater clinical expertise and experience. The student midwives and junior midwives rarely challenged this authority, but used subversive techniques to create a sense of compliance, 'playing the game', where they were attempting to achieve the 'with women' ideology within the 'with institution' environment. This duality of ideology has been seen throughout this book and, despite the highlighting of this phenomenon by the likes of Hunter, it would appear to continue to be problematic.

Student midwives can be seen to be maintaining their personal integrity by playing a part, surface-acting or using display rules (Mann 2004, Hochschild 1983, Goffman 1959). It would appear, though, that these studies of midwives' struggles with their ideology are more similar to the emotional labour described by Hochschild (1979), rather than the emotion work or 'gift' discussed by Hochschild (2003) and Bolton (2000), despite Hunter (2005) labelling it emotion work. It may be that the junior or student midwives expected a reciprocal emotional exchange with their senior colleagues, to allow them to offer the 'gift' to women, as seen previously (Bolton 2000, Hochschild 2003). However this behaviour is interpreted, Hunter (2005) clearly identified the distress it causes those who are caught up in an environment where they are expected to comply with one set of framing and feeling rules, when they feel compelled to adhere to another.

The struggles, identified by Hunter (2005), that were experienced by student midwives and newly qualified midwives, can also be seen as part of the experience of more experienced midwives as well, whether they are working in a hospital setting or the community. Deery (2009) clearly demonstrates that, on top of the need to develop relationships with women and the pressures of large caseloads, midwives need to use extensive emotion work to manage their relationships with each other and to manage the organisational demands.

Hunter continues to explore the emotion work of midwives and, in her study published in 2006, she used an ethnographic approach to develop an understanding of community-based midwives. She focused on their relationship with the women for whom they were caring. This is particularly significant, as national and international policy is to work in partnership with women (ICM 2006, NSF (DoH) 2004, NICE 2003, 2006).

The concept of reciprocity is useful in understanding this relationship between midwives and women (Hunter 2006). Reciprocity can be defined as the sharing, giving and taking of a commodity, as opposed to an altruistic giving without expectation of gain. Reciprocal relationships and interactions have been seen as important in the provision of emotion work, earlier in this chapter, when considering the sharing of gifts between nurses and their colleagues and nurses and patients. For the nurses in Bolton's study (2000), there was an acceptance of giving 'the gift' to patients and their (dead) babies, but there was the need or expectation of a reciprocal relationship with their colleagues. There are those who would suggest no-one actually does anything that is truly altruistic, as it can be seen that, although a giver may not receive anything substantive in return, they may gain an inner sense of self-worth and fulfilment. It could, therefore, be determined that all relationships and interactions are reciprocal at some level.

In Hunter's 2006 study, she identified the strategies used to gain rapport, to build a relationship, such as self-disclosure, humour and teasing. The relationships were emotionally rewarding for the midwives when the women allowed them to exhibit an individualised approach and were receptive to midwifery advice (Hunter 2006). Hunter (2006) identified four key interactional styles: balanced exchange, reverse exchange, rejected exchange and unsustainable exchange.

It is only the balanced exchange, or a reciprocal relationship, that offers a clear, rewarding experience for the midwife; all the others create emotion work for them (Hunter 2006). This is a simplistic model and midwife-woman interactions are more complex, but it can provide a method for further exploration of this complex social process (Hunter 2006). In her later study, Hunter (2009) discussed some of the complexities of these interactions, identifying how as midwives move from one woman and one situation to another, their approach changes.

Women find their relationships with midwives to be of key significance and midwives have the power to mar the woman's experience (Anderson 2000). Interactions vary quite considerably in different situations and with different women. Midwives are suggested to attempt to adjust their behaviour to 'fit' with the woman's, in an attempt to develop a therapeutic or trusting relationship. Indeed, Hunter (2009) labelled this adjusting to situations as the 'mixed messages' that senior midwives sent to student midwives. The junior midwives became confused with the ideological stance, framing and feeling rules they should adopt. When faced with this confusion, these student midwives can be seen to adopt a variety of coping strategies, but predominantly used 'switching off and toughening up', a self- protective approach that may be problematic for providing emotional care. Coping strategies could range from seeking support from others, to more bullying activities.

Hunter (2009) found that offering mixed messages occurred mainly in hospital settings, but Deery (2009) acknowledged similar struggles for community midwives. These messages were labelled affective neutrality and affective awareness. Neutrality is where the midwife does not engage with the situation on an emotional level; they suppress their emotions and behave in a professional manner (Hunter 2009). Emotional awareness is demonstrated by the sharing of emotions and support. These appear closely linked to the ideologies of 'with institution' or 'with profession' and 'with woman'.

Kirkham (2009) acknowledges that women gain their emotional cues from midwives and, if midwives are defensive and self-protective, women will not seek emotional support from them. This may achieve compliance with midwifery services and reduced emotional toll for the midwife, but may also lead to emotional problems for the woman and her baby.

The gift of emotion work is a gift of love; it is something extra, which can be sustained by gratitude and appreciation (Hochschild 2003). It is culturally determined and so gender, social class and power have an impact on what is expected (both display and feeling rules) and culture is always on the move. Cultural changes within our society expect women in the twenty-first century to control their "feelings of fear, vulnerability and the desire to be comforted" (Hochschild 2003:24). Despite this, when a middle-class woman offers comfort by emotion management, traditional views still exist and it is then not appreciated and gratitude is not given, as it is not seen as extra or a gift (Bolton 2000, Hochschild 2003, John and Parsons 2006). There is, though, a positive way forward through midwifery organisational structures, which facilitate the recognition of the importance of the reciprocal relationship where recognition and appreciation can be demonstrated. If a case-loading approach is used, some of the problems are ameliorated (McCourt and Stevens 2009).

It can be seen from Hunter's studies (2001, 2004, 2005, 2006, 2009) that emotion work is widespread in midwifery and can be created by any significant interactions between midwives and others (colleagues or clients). There is general agreement that emotion work is costly, but it is important to ensure quality care (Smith 1992, Bolton 2000, Hunter 2001, 2004, 2005, 2006, 2009, Mann 2004, Deery 2009).

Outcomes for the midwife of offering emotional care

There are three types of emotional outcome between behaviour and feeling: emotional harmony, emotional dissonance and emotional deviance (Mann 2004). Emotional harmony is where the emotion portrayed is the one the person is feeling. Emotional dissonance occurs when feeling rules and organisational rules dictate a person should behave and feel in a certain way, but this is not how the person would like to behave or how they feel. Emotional deviance occurs when the person is expressing their emotions in a way that they feel is appropriate and is the way they feel, but which does not match the organisational rules or expectations. Both emotional dissonance and deviance could cause distress for the carer, whether midwife, nurse or counsellor.

Emotion work can be seen as a double-edged sword, in that it may achieve the necessary outcomes, but it may prove too costly for the psychological wellbeing of the person enacting it. There are studies demonstrating a link between emotional labour stress and 'burn out' (Mann 2004, Sandell 1997) and it may be that, if emotion work is unrecognised, it may incur greater cost, as it is practised in both public and private arenas.

The interactional cognitive phenomenological model of Folkman and Lazarus (1991), could be helpful when trying to establish effective ways of dealing with the stress induced by emotional labour or work (Mann 2004). Some coping strategies for dealing with emotional labour could be strategies such as cognitive restructuring, to acknowledge emotional labour as a high status activity and a skilled part of a person's job. These could be labelled problem-solving, coping strategies. Other coping strategies commonly used for other situations can also be helpful, such as time-out, emotional release, rationalising and humour (Mann 2004). These can be labelled emotion focused coping (Folkman and Lazarus 1991). They may also be useful to help midwives cope with emotion work, or offering the 'gift'.

Summary

Hochschild (1979) offered an early theory of the manipulation of emotions for commercial reasons. This commercialisation, or professional use of emotions, can be seen in healthcare (Smith 1992, Bolton 2000, Mann 2004, 2005, Hunter 2005, 2006). This emotional labour (in the public arena) or emotion work (private arena) can be seen to be a great effort for healthcare professionals, as for the flight attendants in Hochschild's seminal study. Hochschild (2003) and John and Parsons (2006) go on to warn those expecting a manipulation of emotions, particularly emotion work at a deep acting level, in professionals without appreciation and recognition that there may be detrimental effects for those offering this 'gift'.

CHAPTER SEVEN

HOW MIGHT EMOTIONAL SUPPORT HELP WOMEN ON THEIR JOURNEY TO MOTHERHOOD?

Introduction

There is evidence which supports the need for midwives to offer emotionally supportive care for women becoming mothers, to reduce or ameliorate emotional distress. This is to promote the well-being of mother (Barclay et al 1997, Cronin 2003, Miller 2007), baby (Miller et al 1993, Lemaitre-Sillere 1998, McMahon et al 2001) and family (Burke 2003, Tammentie et al 2004a, Tammentie et al 2004b). It is suggested that this can be achieved by facilitating the 'with woman' ideology (Morrissey 2007).

Emotional support

The midwife-woman relationship has been identified as the central element of midwifery care in numerous studies (Fleming 1998b, Fraser1999, Walsh 1999, Pairman 2000, McCourt 2005, Hunter 2006). Researchers have acknowledged that the midwife-woman relationship is essential when supporting women in their transition to motherhood, in becoming mothers (Lundgen 2004). The evidence suggests that the relationship between midwives and women affects the quality of the childbirth experience for women (Anderson 2000, Kitzinger 2006, McCourt et al 2006, Edwards 2009) and that this experience stays with women throughout their lives (Lundgren 2004).

Despite the philosophical emphasis on 'women-centred care' and the need for an intimate relationship between midwife and women, there are some who are cautious of this approach. Carolan and Hodnett (2007) encourage us to reflect on whether this is what women want. They provide evidence that women want the opportunity to engage in the decision-making process, to be provided with consistent, respectful and informative care. The promoters of women-centred intimate care may well respond to this by stating that the relationship they advocate is the best way of achieving what women wanted.

The essential structure of the women's lived experience is one of "wishing for a perfect baby in an altered mode of being, while striving for family communion" (Bondas & Eriksson 2001:835). It could, therefore, be assumed that women would wish to be supported, to achieve their aims of a perfect baby, through their changes in health and being to become a harmonious family. Women appear to need support biologically, emotionally, socially and personally until they have achieved motherhood (Barclay et al 1997, Bondas and Eriksson 2001, Cronin 2003). Achieving motherhood takes time and may not occur until sometime after the baby is born but, with support, women adjust and achieve motherhood (Barclay et al 1997, Bondas and Eriksson 2001, Cronin 2003, Miller 2007).

On the whole, women appear to have unrealistic expectations of themselves and others (Cronin 2003, Miller 2007). This could suggest that midwives need to facilitate more realistic discourses, at the same time as supporting control and confidence. These are not the only psychological needs for women (Barclay et al 1997, Cronin 2003); they can also experience feelings such as loneliness, tearfulness and depression. Indeed, all the above studies exploring the experiences of becoming a mother indicate an emotional struggle with adjustment to motherhood. This could lead to depression and midwives, when they offer emotional support, do so with the intention of preventing or reducing emotional distress and depression.

Postnatal Depression

Maternal depression has been found to have extensive long-term effects on the child (Miller et al 1993, Lemaitre-Sillere 1998, McMahon et al 2001). Whilst the NICE antenatal guidelines (DoH 2003, 2008) do not recommend midwives screen for this, they do indicate midwives should refer those women who have had previous mental health problems to psychiatric services. Nevertheless, the NICE guidelines for postnatal care (DoH 2006) state that midwives should ask about symptoms of depression and, if they linger past day fourteen after the birth, then "urgent action" (DoH 2006:14) should be undertaken.

There is some contention about whether emotional distress around the time of becoming a mother is a 'normal' part of the transition, or whether it is pathological, given that most women experience some emotional lability or 'baby blues' (around 50 – 80% of women) (Evins and Theofastous 1997). The prevalence of depression in a review of recent research was found to be 12.9% during pregnancy and 19.2% postnatal (Gavin et al 2005), with post-partum psychosis affecting less than 1% (Evins and Theofastous1997). These figures may, though, be just the 'tip of the iceberg', if the work of Whitton, Warner and Appleby (1996) is taken into consideration. Their study suggests that, out of the women identified as having problems, only 32% believed that they had postnatal depression and only 12% had spoken to a health-care professional about it. Barclay and Lloyd (1996) suggest that, if the figures are as high as suggested, then postnatal depression is either endemic or that psychiatric labels are being inappropriately applied. Others, such as Lawler and Sinclair (2003), suggest that women need to go through a type of grief process to adjust to a new way of being in a new world and Nicholas (1998) that it may be 'normal' to experience emotional distress.

There has been growing concern for women who experience emotional distress around the birth of their babies, with the Department of Health (1999) highlighting post-natal depression as a priority within the National Service Framework (NSF) for Mental Health, NICE antenatal and postnatal mental health guidance (NICE 2007) and a focus on mental health in the NSF for children, young people and maternity services in England (DoH 2004). Post- natal depression (PND) is a major health concern for many women (Dennis and Kavanagh 2002) and those who care for them and their children. "Taking seriously the woman's experiences and the hidden questions that reveal suffering in both lay and professional caring, might prevent the serious post-partum misery of motherhood" (Bondas and Eriksson 2001: 824). Whatever label is used to identify the woman's experience, becoming a mother is an emotional time (Barclay and Lloyd 1996).

Edinburgh Post Natal Depression Scale

The most extensively used tool to screen for PND is the Edinburgh Post Natal Depression Scale (Cox et al 1987). This is despite other measures that have recently been developed, such as the Post-Partum Screening Scale (PPSS), which has been found to correlate well with both the EPNDS and the Beck Depression Inventory II (BDI II), which is used widely in mental health arenas. However, the PPSS is not widely used at present (Beck and Gable 2001). It has been suggested that the EPNDS is widely validated and reliable (Clifford et al 1999), but it did not meet the criteria of the National Screening Committee (NSC) for acceptance as the national screening tool. Adams (2002) discusses the findings of the NSC and offers a number of reasons why it does not meet their criteria – it is not precise or simple, it is not appropriate or acceptable for all women and it is not a diagnostic test. She also states they suggest it is unethical to screen using this tool if there are not enough resources to provide the necessary care. Despite this, the Community Practitioners and Health Visitors Association continue to recognise the EPNDS as a useful tool, as they identify that there are no others available to them (Adams 2002).

If Beck's Depression Inventory, which has been widely validated for clinical application by psychologists, and the EPNDS are compared, it can be seen there are a number of overlapping elements, such as sadness and crying, but also a number of differences. Despite the usefulness of the Beck's questionnaire, it is not widely available to midwives. Some studies have used other scales, such as the Profile of Mood Status Questionnaire (Hayes et al 2001), Hospital Anxiety and Depression Scale or a psychiatric interview using the Diagnostic Statistical Manual (IV) or International Classification of Diseases (10), all of which are used for other psychiatric disorders.

Although a number of scales have been used, PND has continued to be difficult to predict, with antenatal screening disappointing (Burgha at al 2000). Despite the problems with EPNDS, some of the findings of the studies in which it has been used are very useful for understanding the area, for example, women have been said to score more highly when screened antenatally than postnatally (Evans et al 2001).

Beck (2001) undertook a meta-analysis of the risk factors for PND and found thirteen predictors: prenatal depression, low self- esteem, childcare stress, prenatal anxiety, life stress, lack of social support, marital status, unplanned pregnancy, and socio-economic status. These findings are not particular surprising, as all of these issues could be cited as risk factors for depression, outside of the postpartum period. Beck goes on to suggest that there could be a cumulative effect, leading to overload and depression. Whilst Beck has established a strong link with psychosocial problems, such as poor support, individual social issues, such as debt, have not been determined as individual predictors (Reading and Reynolds 2001).

There have been a number of studies exploring the efficacy of treatment regimes. There is evidence to suggest that a cognitive behavioural approach (CBT) is useful (Prendergast and Autin 2001, Chabrol et al 2002) with social support (Taggart et al 2000), group therapy, (Forrester 2001), hormones (Lawrie et al 2002) and antidepressants (Hoffbrand et al 2002) giving some positive impact. A meta-analysis of treatment for depression during pregnancy and the postpartum period was undertaken by Bledsoe and Grote (2006). They found that, of the 16 interventions compared, 14 of them had a significant positive effect. Medication, medication with CBT, group therapy, interpersonal psychotherapy (IPT) and CBT approaches all had a significance level where the p value was less than 0.001. A psychodynamic or counselling approach to treatment only gained a significance of p as less than 0.014 and an educational approach did not have a significant impact on the women's depression.

Despite the lack of impact of postnatal education on depression, an antenatal educational approach was found to significantly reduce the depression experienced by mothers in a Hong Kong study (Ngai et al 2009). This program, though, could be considered to be using a cognitive approach as it focused on cognitive restructuring, problem solving and efficacy enhancement.

It is clear that there are many effective treatment approaches available to women with postnatal depression. Despite the evidence to support effective interventions, a clear treatment regime has not been identified. It is acknowledged that PND is eminently treatable (Dennis and Kavanagh 2001), leading to the suggestion that resources are focused on treating the woman after onset, rather than on recognition and prevention (Hayes et al 2001). This is in contrast to the suggestions of Evans et al (2001), who identified that antenatal depression is more severe that postnatal depression and should therefore be the focus of research.

Judy Shakespear (2001) wrote a detailed report for the NSC, covering the features, impact, treatment and screening for PND. She suggested that there is no evidence that primary prevention is useful, that current antenatal classes are ineffective and that midwives and health visitors do not receive appropriate education. Barclay et al (1997) and Bondas and Eriksson (2001) also identify the ineffectiveness of antenatal care and Mac Arthurs et al (2002) goes on to suggest that postnatal care, offered to mothers, does not address their mental health issues.

The government in the UK, as part of the changes in the NHS in the latter stage of the last century, introduced the National Institute for Clinical Excellence which has now become the National Institute for Health and Clinical Excellence. This organisation advises governmental policies and the NHS in care provision. The NICE guidelines for the routine postnatal care of women and their babies (2006) and the NICE guidelines for routines care for healthy pregnant women (2003, 2008) have sought to offer guidance to those caring for women at this time, after weighing up the available research and economic variables. The antenatal guidelines (NICE 2003, 2008) after a consideration of the evidence, some of which has already been provided here, lead midwives not to routinely screen women, during pregnancy, to predict postnatal depression and not to offer antenatal education interventions to reduce perinatal or postnatal depression. They do, though, state that midwives should refer women who have experienced previous mental illness for a psychiatric assessment.

This may be due to the previous studies focusing on midwife- led antenatal classes and, as suggested by Shakespear (2001), midwives may not be educated to provide the type of psycho-education given in Ngai et al's (2009) study. NICE also consider the economics of healthcare provision and, as stated by Shakespear (2001), if there are not the resources to provide the identified care needs of women at this time, then it is unethical to screen for it.

In contrast, one of the priorities, in the postnatal period, in the NICE guidelines (2006) states that "At each postnatal contact, women should be asked about their emotional well-being, what family and social support they have and usual coping strategies for dealing with day- to- day matters. Women and their families/partners should be encourages to tell their healthcare professional about any changes in mood, emotional state and behaviour that are outside of the woman's normal pattern" (NICE 2006: 6). Given that women in some studies report higher levels of mental distress in pregnancy (Evans et al 2001), the focus on mental well-being in the postnatal period and the avoidance of approaching the topic of mental well-being in the antenatal period, is somewhat surprising. Treatment efficacy and costs (Dennis and Kavanagh 2001, Hayes et al 2001) may have had an impact on this decision.

However the emotional distress is labelled, if emotionally supportive care can prevent or reduce its occurrence and does not require additional resources, it would appear prudent to offer this type of care, given the impact on mother, child and family. Certainly, the midwives in my study appeared to believe emotional support can alleviate emotional distress. Morrissey (2007) goes on to encourage midwives in their 'with woman' emotional approach to care to facilitate mental well-being. Barclay and Lloyd (1996) identify that becoming a mother is a huge transition involving physiological, psychological and social reorganisation. All transitions take some time to achieve adjustment, but the transition to motherhood involves a change in assumptions about the world and an acceptance that the transition is lifelong.

Becoming a mother can include feeling drained, unready and alone and involve some sense of loss. Loss of previous relationships with partners and friends, loss of lifestyle, time, freedom and confidence can all be part of the experience (Barclay et al 1997). Women who experience this loss as distress also experience unsettled behaviour in their babies (McMahon et al 2001). For some women, these feelings dissipate over a short period of time, but for others they can take months to overcome. This occurs at a time when a woman is expected to feel full of joy as a result of her baby (Barclay et al 1997).

The emotional distress felt by mothers has been found to have long-lasting effects on the baby or young child. Given the infant's extreme dependence on the mother and their sensitivity to interpersonal contacts, the emotional distress of mothers can have a profound impact on the infant (Murray and Cooper 1997). Cognitive development of these young children can be significantly impaired, in comparison to those children whose mothers who do not experience distress. When the infants of distressed mothers were assessed for their interpersonal functioning, they were found to have a lower rate of interaction, poorer concentration and less effective sharing, and to engage in more negative responses. They were also less sociable to strangers.

Attachment issues

Studies of attachment behaviours demonstrated more children of distressed mothers to be insecurely attached (Murray and Cooper 1997, Logsdon et al 2003). These children were also more likely to have behavioural problems. These findings fit well with the theoretical work of Bowlby and the experimental studies of Ainsworth (Papalia et al 1998).

Attachment is where the infant and mother are in a continuous relationship, where the infant experiences warmth and intimacy and both find satisfaction and enjoyment (Bowlby 1951). This theory of attachment developed over a number of years and in 1973, a model of how a lack of early attachment could have long-term effects on the person was presented (Papalia et al 1998). This was called the internal working model. This suggested that early life experiences lead the infant to develop beliefs and expectations about the world and relationships. If the infant has received continuous love from its mother it will develop the belief that people can be trusted, that they are worthy of love and that people care. The infant then carries this forward to future relationships, including their own parenting. These expectations lead to a perception of the world as being benevolent, which is self-reinforcing.

An assessment strategy was developed to measure attachment, called "The Strange Situation" (Ainsworth and Wittig 1969). Three types of attachment: type A labelled "anxious – avoidant attachment", type B labelled "securely attached" and type C labelled "anxious – resistant" were found. Most children were securely attached, but those who were not could go on to have problems throughout their lives, not only with relationships, but in all areas of their development.

A longitudinal study was conducted, comparing the five-year-old children of a group of women who experienced postnatal depression, with a group of well women (Sinclair and Murray 1998). The children of the women who had experienced some level of distress, which was labelled postnatal depression, were found to have difficulty adjusting to school. Whilst this was more problematic for boys in both groups and those with lower socio-economic status, there was a raised level of disturbance in the children whose mothers had experienced depression. There were also higher levels of aggression expressed in children exposed to maternal depression (Hipwell et al 2005).

Evidence consistently demonstrates that the infants and children of women with high levels of distress go on to have developmental and behavioural problems (Miller et al 1993, Lemaitre-Sillere 1998, McMahon et al 2001). It has also been found that a mother with postnatal depression can have an impact on the whole family (Burke 2003, Tammentie et al 2004a, Tammentie et al 2004b).

Mediating factors for this distress were: the nature of the mother baby interactions, prior experience with other people's babies and the nature of the support available to the mother (Barclay et al 1997). Some of the women identified their mothers as their most important support, but the support offered by midwives and nurses was mixed. Postnatal emotional support from the woman's partner was also found to reduce the experience of depression (Lemola et al 2007).

The implications would appear to be that midwives and nurses should be educated to assist women integrate and resolve their labour experiences and realise the magnitude of the changes a new mother faces (Barclay et al 1997). The NICE guidelines for postnatal care direct midwives to not use formal debriefing techniques after the birth, but encourage midwives to check for signs of mental ill health (DoH 2006). Some women need additional emotional and practical support and midwives need to recognise the impact of the individual's social circumstances (Barclay et al 1997). Morrissey (2007) would agree with Barclay et al's recommendations, particularly facilitating midwives to recognise the enormity of the transition for women, but he states that 'being with women' through the transition is the most helpful way to promote their mental health.

The 'with woman' ideology of midwifery and 'women centred' philosophy, stated in government and professional body guidance for midwives, is the approach necessary for managing and reducing emotional distress (Morrissey 2007).

There is limited literature on how midwives provide emotional support to women, despite the apparent need for this type of care. This book has tried to address this issue and in chapters 4 and 5 offers a detailed discussion of the emotional care that midwives offer and the context in which they offer it. It has been seen that, when offering emotional support, midwives do this within what has been labelled the 'with woman' philosophy and, as indicated above, this would appear to be the most appropriate methodology for this type of care.

The midwives in my study, when offering emotional support, appear to be seeking to achieve comfort for the women, or an inner sense of peace. Comfort can be seen to be what most health care professionals seek to facilitate for those in distress.

Comfort

Despite the lack of clarity over the term "support" and other terms such as "emotional support", "therapeutic emotional labour" or "emotional care" within most of the literature available, the enactment of all these terms seems to be aiming for the same goal. The goal would appear to be for emotional well-being and comfort in the woman (NMC 2004).

Comfort is an area in which literature from nursing is more readily available, although there have been a number of studies in midwifery considering the goal of comfort for women in labour. "Comfort is a concept that involves the enhancement of strength and health……. Comfort may be considered the ultimate state of health and therefore may be viewed as the goal of nursing" (Morse et al 1995: 19).

The Nursing and Midwifery Council (2009) states that midwives should provide care for the women and families they work with and they define care as providing help and comfort. This could be seen as a circular discussion; midwives need to provide care, which is comfort, and to achieve comfort they provide care. Therefore a more detailed examination is needed.

Despite comfort being difficult to define, there being a number of theoretical approaches to understanding it, Morse et al (1994) have offered an insight into this concept. They said "Comfort, paradoxically, appears to be a state of embodiment that is beyond awareness, and comfort is best recognised when the patient first leaves the state of discomfort" (Morse et al 1994: 190). They explain that comfort comes from the Latin word *confortare*, which means to strengthen. From their study they identify that patient comfort is linked with strengthening or empowering the person, in relation to their body.

Nursing literature (Morse et al 1994) suggests suffering causes the person to focus on the corporeal, comfort allows the person space to focus on other areas of their lives. Comfort from a midwifery perspective appears to involve mind (psychological), body (corporeal) and spirit (soul) (Schuiling and Sampselle 1999). A state of comfort in the mind involves a feeling of peace and security, freedom from anxiety or worry. Within the body it involves physical needs being met, such as hunger, thirst, sleep, air and freedom from illness. Spiritual comfort involves a feeling of hope and expectation, transcendence from pain and being at one with one's god

(Schuiling and Sampselle 1999). When offering emotional support, midwives appear to aim to facilitate comfort in the women on their journey to motherhood. Their interventions to achieve this appear to correspond well with the literature available on how people need this to be offered to them (Schuiling and Sampselle 1999, Morse 2000, Williams and Irurita 2004).

Discomfort can be considered to be a mostly corporeal experience (Morse et al 1994), but some suggest it has mind, body and spiritual elements (Schuiling and Sampselle 1999). A person's experience of their body when well or comfortable is limited, but when in discomfort this changes (Morse et al 1994). Nine themes of discomfort have been found: dis-eased body, disobedient body, deceiving body, vulnerable body, violated body, enduring body, betraying body, resigned body and betraying mind. This was established by interviewing patients who had experienced extreme pain or discomfort and traumatic injuries or life-threatening illness. Through these interviews, it was explored how the patient gained comfort within each of the nine areas (Morse et al 1994).

One of the themes in Morse et al's (1994) study was the dis-eased body. In this theme, comfort was gained from information about the illness and a belief in the caregiver's ability to provide appropriate care. Within this ill or 'diseased body' theme (Morse et al 1994), in the midwifery situation this may be related to emotional and or physical pain, where suffering seems to take control of the person's whole being. For the sufferer at this time, to regain some understanding of their body offered them some comfort. The control and information-giving apparently sought, and provided by the midwives in my study for the women they care for, would also have an impact on the comfort experienced (Morse et al 1994, Schuiling and Sampselle 1999, Williams and Irurita 2004).

Information-giving is a key element of midwives' role and was discussed in detail in chapter 4 and mentioned in chapter 5. Both Williams and Irurita (2004) and Schuiling and Sampselle (1999) highlighted information-giving as an element of providing comfort. They also recognised the need for those being cared for to feel confident in their caregiver's ability to provide that care. McCourt et al (2000) established that women within midwifery care also needed to be able to trust and have confidence in their midwives. The midwives' role is to facilitate confidence and increase the ability of the women they care for (Kirkham 1999).

Confidence and trust can be seen to be closely related and the words have been used interchangeably when discussing care. Women need to be able to trust the midwives and this trust will give them the confidence that their care needs will be addressed. One of the aims within midwifery is to develop confidence in the women; not only confidence that their care needs will be addressed, but also that women will have confidence in their own ability to care for themselves and their baby.

Roach developed a theory of caring, she was influenced by the philosophical approach of phenomenology, particularly Heidegger, and she also had a clear focus on theology (McCance et al 1999). Roach identified that caring is not unique to nursing but is unique within nursing, which has also been said of midwifery (Lundgren 2004). She conceptualises caring in her 'five Cs': compassion, competence, confidence, conscience and commitment (McCance 1991). This confidence and competence can be seen to closely link to providing the comfort indicated above and can be seen as a core element of care which is central to what a midwife does.

Women do not always feel confident in midwifery services, but it would appear to be important to emotionally support women to achieve comfort. One of the midwives in my study described how she had worked with the woman to develop a trusting relationship using her information-giving, self-disclosure and communication skills. Using her emotion work and emotional support, including gaining trust and confidence, Emily said the woman was "*Much more relaxed, less tearful*" and went on to have a good birth experience.

Morse et al (1994) stress it is not the activity of care that is important, it is the way in which it is undertaken. If it is undertaken 'for' and 'with' the person, instead of 'to' the person, it restores their integrity and assists in moving them towards recovery. This would also appear to be the aim of women-centred care in midwifery. The midwives appear to be aiming to work 'for' and 'with' the women they were caring for. An example from my study is where Diane was working 'for' and 'with' the woman to overcome some of her struggles. She said,

> "We um talked it through to deal with that and um we talked through coping with the baby being awake at night and tips for that, just sitting and talking about getting enough sleep and making sure she was getting enough sleep during the day time".

The 'vulnerable body', another of Morse et al's themes (1994), is seen in situations where pain, or the anticipation of pain, becomes all- consuming. Certainly the midwives in my study recognised vulnerability in the women they were caring for and this led them to offer emotional support.

Comfort at times of vulnerability is gained from feeling safe, secure and trusting in the caregiver. Midwives seek to develop trusting, therapeutic relationships with the women for whom they cared. When the anticipation of pain cannot be removed, the caregiver can offer comfort by protecting, bolstering and advocating for the person (Morse et al 1994). Again, each of these can be found in the midwives' descriptions in my study. Hetty described how she protected the young woman from being in uncomfortable situations (protecting), Diane described reassuring the mother that, as mother, she knew her baby (bolstering) and Hetty needed to advocate for the woman with other professionals.

Another of the nine themes is the violated body. There are times when a person needs to have interventions or examinations that are considered to violate the body. People can comfort themselves at these times by distancing themselves from their bodies (Morse et al 1994). The presence of, and connection with, a caregiver can aid this, by allowing the person to feel safe and secure enough to relinquish part of their body for a short while. Nurses achieve this connection by their use of their hands, eyes and voices (Morse et al 1994). There are times when a person knows that they cannot remove themselves from their discomfort and have to endure it, which is another of the identified themes. Comfort was gained at this time by refocusing attention on something that offered hope.

The resigned body occurs when the body has permanently changed and the person needs to come to terms with this, to achieve comfort using a tolerance of self and keeping going. Although women in their transition to motherhood would not immediately be considered to be suffering, for many this is how it feels (Barclay et al 1996). For these women, they need to come to terms with a permanently changed body and the other changes associated with that. For women experiencing suffering in this way, they need to accept their changed way of being to gain comfort. It is an acceptance of oneself and ones limitations. The midwives in my study can be seen to be attempting to guide the women towards this acceptance of their new way of being, by helping them to negotiate managing their day-to- day activities and recognising the normality of their experiences. Carol said,

> "I think really we need to make them feel they are normal and are not abnormal in any way; that this is normal".

The last three of Morse's themes focus on the body and mind betraying the person. The deceiving body is where the person feels well, but actually the body is deteriorating. The person can be comforted here by recognising that this is a normal function of bodies, or by having check-ups and tests to demonstrate that the body is not deteriorating in an excessive manner. The betraying body occurs when the person believes that they are coping well but their body is showing signs of a lack of coping. This can occur in less noticeable ways, such as appearing tired, but may occur in psychosomatic illness, such as heart attacks and migraine. Comfort could be gained in these situations by raising the person's awareness and facilitating their acceptance of appropriate help, such as counselling and relaxation exercises (Morse et al 1994).

Women experience pain in childbirth and for some this is experienced as extreme suffering, and the understanding of suffering and comfort from the above nursing perspective is useful for the midwife to understand. Comfort can enhance the ability to cope with great pain and empower women (Schuiling and Sampselle 1999). To participate in decision-making, to plan and feel in control, will enhance the comfort felt by women at this time. To have control is a concept that occurs frequently in midwifery literature (DoH 1993, Levy 1999a,b,c, DoH 2004, McCourt 2005). In the literature on comfort, such as Morse et al (1994) and Williams and Irurita (2004), control is also described as a means of facilitating comfort.

Other theoretical approaches to comfort include the idea that, to facilitate comfort, the comforter needs to "provide support, relieve pain and anxiety, communicating, using touch and comforting family and friends" (Schuiling and Sampselle 1999: 79). Touching and talking are the main components of facilitating comfort and listening is important for the most distressed (Schuiling and Sampselle 1999). These behaviours also link well with the findings and theory of Morse (2001, 2000). She would agree that touching and talking are major elements in attempting to facilitate comfort and with those who have lost control, she identified nurses use "comfort talk register, eye contact and touch" (Morse 2001: 52).

Research pertaining to comfort in childbearing is scarce and, despite comfort meaning more to women than elimination of pain, the limited publications available were focused on this (Schuiling and Sampselle

1999). The elimination of pain has been the focus of the medical profession to achieve comfort, but this limits the understanding of suffering and comfort (Morse 2001). Comfort for women appeared to include reduction of tiredness, not being hungry and a feeling of being relaxed (Schuiling and Sampselle 1999); this has been acknowledged throughout the centuries (Rhodes 1995). Women also sought a supportive presence and a caring approach, which could be considered to be the same as Morse et al's (1994) statement of the need for presence and connection.

Midwifery and nursing theoretical approaches to suffering and comfort are very similar, despite their differing focus (Morse et al 1994, 1995, Schuiling and Sampselle 1999, Morse 2000, 2001). Morse and her colleagues (1994, 1995, 2000, 2001) focused on developing a theory of suffering and comfort, gained from the experiences of patients and nurses. Schuiling and Sampselle (1999) focused on identifying the activities of midwives in their attempts to facilitate comfort for women during childbirth. Elements of Morse's (2000, 2001) enduring and emotional suffering can be seen in Schuiling and Sampselle's (1999) paper and in my study.

The opportunity to gain some control over themselves or their environment facilitated a sense of comfort for some people (Morse et al 1994). Facilitating choice and control are key issues in midwifery care, in line with government directives (particularly Changing Childbirth - DoH 1993). The midwives in my study also appeared to be attempting to facilitate control in the women they were caring for. Gina said,

> "I felt I was making her feel that she was in control and trying to accommodate her wishes".

This was done to reduce emotional distress and increase comfort for the women. It is generally assumed that to have information allows for informed choices and a feeling of control, which is advocated by both midwifery literature (Kirkham et al 2002a) and government policy (DoH 1993).

The midwives in my study undertook home-visiting when they perceived the women needed emotional support. The reasons offered for home-visiting were that it facilitated relationship development; it allowed women to be more comfortable and moved the perceived power from the midwife, giving control to the woman.

All the areas highlighted as important for facilitating comfort within the person (Morse et al 1994, Schuiling and Sampselle 1999, Williams and Irurita 2004) have been seen in the descriptions from the midwives in my study, when they were offering emotionally supportive care. These activities included giving information, control, developing trust along with the communication skills of touch, voice and eye contact to focus the women. Midwives can therefore be assumed by their words and experiences to be seeking to induce comfort in the women for whom they are caring.

Normality to develop comfort

Normality was an area discussed in chapter 4 as important in the emotional care of women on their journey to motherhood. The midwives in my study identified the need to allow the women to have a sense of normality to create comfort in them. They felt it was important that the women should feel that their experiences were normal and the midwives also tried to encourage the women to believe that their births were normal. Carol said,

> "I think really we need to make them feel they are normal and are not abnormal in any way; that this is normal".

John and Parsons' (2006) study provided the women's perspective on the importance of being treated as if they were normal and the midwives behaving as if they were having normal conversations. The midwives in their study also identified that they were trying to ensure the experience was normal for the women. The experience of being 'normal' appears to have a duality of meaning within midwifery, in that the midwives appear to try to facilitate a 'normal birth' and the experience of 'being normal' also appears to mean the woman not being distressed or believing that there is anything wrong with her. They appear to use both meanings of normal and attempt to achieve both types of normality to facilitate the women gaining comfort (Morse et al 1994).

It is again difficult to know if the midwives hold the belief that they should encourage the sense of normality because they are led to do so by government guidelines, or whether there is another ideological reason for this. The 'with woman' ideology supports the belief that becoming a mother is a normal process, not a medical condition requiring intervention. This is an ideological standpoint that is being increasingly promoted by government as well as midwives (NSF – DoH 2004).

A feeling of control to facilitate comfort

The midwives in my study could be seen to promote a feeling of control, as identified above, to allow the women to feel they had some command over what may feel like a time of chaos and powerlessness.

Control, though, appears to be a somewhat illusory thing and there are a number of papers in the literature focusing on control within midwifery (Lomax and Robinson 1996, Fleming 1998a,b, Levy 1998a,b,c,d, Walsh 1999, Green et al 2000, McCourt 2005). This appears to be mostly due to the call for continuity, control and choice in midwifery through documents like Changing Childbirth (DoH 1993). Some studies suggest women are gaining control in midwifery and, in doing, are creating extra problems for midwives. Fleming (1998b) found that some women are assertively making demands and taking control, which has coerced midwives to take on work that overloads them. There was no indication from the midwives' descriptions in my study that they felt coerced into providing extra care. Despite this, Emily did feel that the women she was caring for had unrealistic expectations of the midwifery service, which created the woman's initial distress. Emily said,

> "But for some reason she felt she had been let down by the system because she had been seen by 2 different midwives, she hadn't taken into account that she had.... Moved"... "She got herself in a terrible state about it".

Some studies suggest all the control lies with the midwives (Lomax and Robinson 1996, Levy 1998c), whilst others state that women and midwives have no control - it is all in the hands of medicine and the managers (Kirkham et al 2002). Levy's (1998d,e) work would paint the picture of control not belonging to anyone; it is taken, given and passed around like some high-stakes, complex game. Perhaps the best that midwives can achieve is the 'feeling of control', for themselves and the women for whom they care, as that is all that is available within the complexities of the current culture (see chapter 5 for a discussion of the culture within which midwifery sits).

Interestingly, the comfort the midwives are seeking to achieve, by offering emotionally supportive care, is said to facilitate a feeling of control in the women for whom they are caring (Schuiling and Sampselle 1999). This may lead to the conclusion that, if midwives focus on their supportive skills, there will be little need for them to advocate for women and empower them.

As was highlighted previously, facilitating control in those suffering can produce a sense of comfort (Morse et al 1994) and the midwives in my study can be seen to be trying to achieve this, despite enacting protective steering (Levy 1998c).

Issues raised

This discussion facilitates an understanding that the midwives perform an important role in the emotional care of women on their journey to motherhood. The emotional support they offer women is intended to reduce emotional distress and provide comfort. This has been acknowledged through both nursing and midwifery literature. There are, though, a couple of areas of concern in the literature available. The first is information-giving. Midwives in my recent study indicate that they may continue to be enacting 'protective steering' but, despite this not being the recommended approach, from the descriptions of these midwives, is it undertaken in the best interests of the women. The midwives may, though, be criticised for using this approach, as it can be seen to reduce the woman's ability to make informed decisions and access control. It could also be suggested that they are managing the information- giving and maintaining an element of control, instead of facilitating empowerment and control in the women.

The maintenance of control by midwives may also reduce the comfort that is achieved, given the literature on gaining comfort. This does not appear to be the perception of the midwives, though. The midwives in my study believed, given the positive emotional expressions by the women they were caring for, that they have facilitated comfort and safe motherhood by reducing distress.

The other area of concern, arising from this exploration of the emotional care of midwives, is the emotion work undertaken by them. The midwives in my study, appear to be offering women the 'gift' of emotional support, which has an associated emotional toll. For some of them this is ameliorated by close relationships with their colleagues or the woman and her family, and encouragement and endorsement from them. This could be seen in the circle of care described in chapter 4. The colleagues and families offered the appreciation and recognition needed to support midwives in their emotion work. Sadly, some midwives still experience limited support in their emotional care, leading to increased emotion work which can lead to stress and 'burn out' in them (Sandell 1997, Mann 2004). This could be particularly seen in Hetty, one of the midwives in my study. Hetty appeared to have little support and increased stress placed on her by other professionals. In fact, it can be seen that all the midwives in my study are trying to behave in a 'with woman' manner, at the same time as trying to adhere to the 'being professional / with institution' approach. This working with opposing or divergent ideologies can increase the emotion work and stress for midwives.

Summary

Women are at risk of becoming emotionally distressed during pregnancy and as new mothers. This distress may be seen in many guises from the odd tearful moment through to postpartum psychosis. This distress, if it leads to poor mother-baby interactions and insecure attachment, can have long term effects on the child. The midwives in my study appear to come alongside women, enacting the 'with woman' philosophy of care to offer emotional support. This 'with woman' approach is said to be helpful in facilitating emotional wellbeing (Morrissey 2007).

Emotional support may, therefore, be considered to help women on their journey to motherhood by offering them some comfort at a time of emotional turmoil, protecting their emotional wellbeing and in turn enhancing their ability to interact with their babies.

REFERENCES

Adams, C., 2002. Use of the Edinburgh Post Natal Depression Screening Scale. *Community Practitioner*, 75 (4), 142-143.

Ainsworth, M., Wittig, B.A., 1969. Attachment and exploratory behaviour of one year olds in a strange situation. *In*: Foss B.M. ed. *Determinants of Infant Behaviour.* Vol. 4 London: Methuen.

Anderson, T., 2000. Feeling safe to let go: The relationship between a woman and her midwife during second stage of labour. *In*: Kirkham, M., ed. *The Midwife-mother relationship.* London: MacMillan Press Ltd. 92-118.

Atkinson, B., 2006. Gaining Motherhood, losing identity? *MIDIRS Midwifery Digest,* 16 (2), 170-174.

Ball, J.A., 1994. *Reaction to Motherhood, The role of postnatal care,* 2nd ed. revised and enlarged. Cheshire: Elsevier, Books for Midwives.

Barclay, L., Everitt, L., Rogan, T., Schmied, V., Wyllie, A., 1997. Becoming a mother – an analysis of women's experience of early motherhood. *Journal of Advanced Nursing,* 25, 719-728.

Barclay, L., Lloyd, B., 1996. The misery of motherhood: alternative approaches to maternal distress. *Midwifery,* 12, 136-139.

Barker, S., 2007. *Vital notes for nurses: psychology.* Oxford: Blackwell Science.

Barnes, D.L., Balber, L.G. 2007. *The Journey to Parenthood, myths, reality and what really matters.* Oxford: Radcliffe Publishing.

Beck, C.T., 2001. Predictors of Postpartum Depression, an update. *Nursing Research* vol 50 no. 5.

Begbie, L., 2004. Midwifery: A mother's perspective. *Midwifery Matters.* Winter Issue 103.

Bledsoe, S.E., Grote, N.K., 2006. Treating Depression During Pregnancy and the Postpartum: A Preliminary Meta-Analysis. *Research on Social Work Practice.* Vol 16 No 2 109-120

Bolton, S.C., 2000. Who cares? Offering emotion work as a 'gift' in the nursing labour process. *Journal of Advanced Nursing*, 32 (3), 580-586.

Bondas, T., Eriksson, K., 2001. Women's lived experiences of pregnancy: A tapestry of joy and suffering. *Qualitative Health Research,* 11 (6), 824-840.

Bone, D., 2009. Epidurals not Emotions: the care deficit in US Maternity Care. *In*: Hunter, B., Deery, R., *Emotions in Midwifery and Reproduction*. Hampshire: Palgrave MacMillan, 56-73.

Bowlby, J., 1951. Maternal care and mental health. *Bulletin of the World Health Organisation*, 3, 355-535.

—. 1969. *Attachment and loss: separation*. New York: Basic books.

Brown, S., Small, R., Lumley, J., 1997. Being a 'Good Mother'. *Journal of Reproductive & Infant Psychology*, 15 (2) May.

Burke, L., 2003. The impact of maternal depression on familial relationships. *International Review of Psychiatry*, 15, 243-255.

Burnard, P., 2002. *Learning Human Skills, an experiential and reflective guide for nurses and health care professionals*, 4th ed. Oxford: Butterworth Heinemann.

Butler, M.M., Fraser, D.M., Murphy, R.J.L., 2008. What are the essential competencies required of a midwife at the point of registration? *Midwifery*, 24 (3), 260-269.

Callister, L.C., Freeborn, D., 2007. Nurse Midwives with Women: Ways of Knowing in Nurse Midwives. *International Journal for Human Caring*, 11 (1), 8-15.

Campbell, A.V., 1984. *Moderated Love, A Theology of Professional Care*. London: SPCK.

Cappuccini. G., Cochrane, R., 2000. Life with the first baby: women's satisfaction with the division of roles. *Journal of Reproductive and Infant Psychology*. Vol. 18, No 3, 189-202.

Carolan, M., Hodnett, E., 2007. 'With woman' philosophy: examining the evidence, answering the questions. *Nursing Inquiry*, 14 (2), 140-152.

Carper, B.A., 1978. Fundamental patterns of knowing in nursing. *Advances in Nursing Science*, 1 (1), 13-23.

Cattrell, R., Lavender, T., Wallymahmed, A., Kingdon, C., Riley, J., 2005. Postnatal care: what matters to midwives. *British Journal of Midwifery*, 13 (4), 206-213.

Cohen, J.,A., 1991. Two portraits of caring: a comparison of the artists, Leininger and Watson. *Journal of Advanced Nursing*, 16, 899-909.

Coupland, J., Coupland, N., Robinson, J. D. 1992. "How are you?" Negotiating phatic communication. *Language in Society*, 21, 207-230.

Cox, A.D., Puckering, C., Bond, A., Mills, M. 1987. The impact of maternal depression in young children. *Journal of Child Psychology and Psychiatry*, 28, 917-928.

Cronin, C., 2003. First-time mothers – identifying their needs, perceptions and experiences. *Journal of Clinical Nursing*, 12, 260-267.

Davies, M., 2002. *The Blackwell Companion to Social Work.* Oxford: Blackwell Publishing

Dennis, C.L., Kavanagh, J., 2001. Psychosocial Interventions for Preventing Post Partum Depression. *The Cochrane Collaboration*: Wiley Publishers. www.thecochranelibrary.com

Department of Health, 1993. *Changing Childbirth, report from the expert maternity group.* London: HMSO.

—. 1997. *The New NHS – Modern, Dependable.* London: The stationery office.

—. 1998. NHS Executive. *A First-Class Service.* Leeds: Department of Health.

—. 1999. *National Service Framework for Mental Health.* London: HMSO.

—. 2000. *The NHS Plan: A plan for investment, a plan for reform: a summary.* London: HMSO.

—. 2004. National Service Framework for children, young people and maternity services in England. London: The Stationary office.

—. 2007. *Good Practice in Learning Disability Nursing.* www.dh.gov.uk/publications

—. 2009. Valuing People Now. London: The stationary Office

—. 2010. White Paper, *Equity and Excellence; liberating the NHS.* London: MH Government

Devane, D., 1996. Sexuality and midwifery. *British Journal of Midwifery,* 4 (8), 414-420.

Diemer, G.A. 1997. Expectant Fathers: Influence of Perinatal Education on Stress, Coping and Spousal Relations. *Research in Nursing & Health*, 20, 281-293

DiQuinzio, P., 1999. *The Impossibility of Motherhood, feminism, individualism, and the problem of mothering.* London: Routledge.

Doggett, C., Burrett, S., Osburn, D.A., 2007. *Home visiting during pregnancy and after birth for women with an alcohol or drug problem (review).* The Cochrane Collaboration: Wiley Publishers. www.thecochranelibrary.com

Downe, S., 2006. Engaging with the concept of unique normality in childbirth. *British Journal of Midwifery*, 1 (6), 352-356.

Drife, J., 2004. *Why Mothers die: the sixth report of the confidential enquiries into maternal deaths in the United Kingdom.* London: RCOG Press.

Dunn-Toroosian, V. 2003. The Family, chapter 4. In Squire, C. *The Social Context of Birth.* Oxford: Radcliffe Medical Press.

Edwards, N.P., 2000. Women Planning Homebirths: Their own views on their Relationships with Midwives. *In*: Kirkham, M., ed. *The Midwife-Mother Relationship*. Hampshire: Palgrave MacMillan, 55-84.

Egan, G., 1977. *The skilled helper*. Monterey, CA: Brooks/Cole.

Evans, J., Heron, J., Francomb, H., Oke, S., Golding, J., 2001. Cohort study of depressed mood during pregnancy after child birth. *British Medical Journal,* 323 (4th August), 257-260.

Engqvist, I., Ahlin, A., Ferszt, G., Nilsson, K. 2010. Nurses – Psychiatrist' main collaborators when treating women with postpartum psychosis. *Journal of Psychiatric and Mental Health Nursing*. 17, 494-502

Evins, G., Theofrastous, J., 1997. Post partum depression: a review of post partum screening. *Primary Care Update Ob/Gyns,* 4 (6), 241-6.

Exley, H., 2004. *Mum*. Herts; Helen Exley gift books.

Field, T., Healy, B., Goldstein, S., Perry, S., Bendell, D., Schanberg, S., Zimmerman, E.A., Kuhn, C., 1988. Infants of depressed mothers show "depressed" behaviour even with nondepressed adults. *Child Development*, 59, 1569-1579.

Fletcher, R., 2009. Promoting Infant Well-Being in the Context of Maternal Depression by Supporting the Father. *Infant Mental Health Journal.* Vol. 30, no 1, 95-102

Fleming, V.E.M., 1998a. Women-with-midwives-with-women: a model of interdependence. *Midwifery,* 14, 137-143.

—. 1998b. Women and midwives in partnership: a problematic relationship*? Journal of Advanced Nursing,* 27, 8-14.

Folkman, S., Lazarus, R.S., 1991. The concept of coping. *In:* Monat, A., Lazarus, R.S., eds. *Stress and Coping: an anthology*, 3rd ed. New York: Columbia University Press.

Fraser, D.M., 1999. Women's perceptions of Midwifery Care: A longitudinal study to shape curriculum development. *Birth,* 26 (2), 99-107.

Fraser, D.M., Cooper, M.A., 2003. *Myles Textbook for Midwives*, 14th ed. London: Churchill Livingstone.

Freshwater, D., Stickley, T., 2004. The Heart of the art: emotional intelligence in nurse education. *Nursing Inquiry,* 11 (2), 91-98.

—. 2005. Action research for changing and improving practise. *In*: Holloway, I., ed. *Qualitative Research in Health Care*. Berkshire: Open University Press.

Fullerton, D., 1997. Preventing and reducing the adverse effects teenage pregnancy. *Health Visitor* 70 (5), 197-199.

Gavin, N.I., Gaynes, B.N., Lohr, K.N., Meltzer-Brody, S., Gartlehner, G., Swinson, T. 2005. Perinatal depression: A systematic review of prevalence and incidence. *Obstetrics and Gynaecology*, 106, 1071-1083

Gee, C.B., McNerney, C.M., Reiter, M.J., Leaman S.C. 2007. Adolescant and Young Adult Mother's Relationship Quality During the Transition to Parenthood: Associations with Father Involvement in Fragile Families. *Journal Youth Adolescence*. 36, 213-224

General Social Care Council, 2010. Codes of Practice for Social Care Workers. www.gscc.org.uk

Giorgi, A., 1997a. The Theory, Practice, and Evaluation of The Phenomenological Method as a Qualitative Research Procedure. *Journal of Phenomenological Psychology*, 28 (2), 235-260.

—. 1997b. The Theory, Practice, and Evaluation of The Phenomenological Method as a Qualitative Research Procedure. *Journal of Phenomenological Psychology*, 28 (2), 235-260.

Goffman, E., 1959. *The Presentation of Self in everyday Life*. London: Penguin Books.

—. 1970. *Strategic Interaction*. Oxford: Blackwell Publishing.

Gross, R,. 2001. *Psychology. The science of mind and behaviour*, 4th ed. London: Hodder and Stoughton.

Green, J. M., Kafetsios, K., 1997. Positive experiences of early motherhood: predictive variables from a longitudinal study. *Journal of Reproductive and Infant Psychology*, 15 (2), 141-157.

Hall, J., 2001. *Midwifery, Mind and Spirit, emerging issues of care*. Oxford: Elsevier, Books for midwives.

—. 2002. Understanding sexuality in midwifery practice. *Midwifery today – international midwife*, Summer page 47.

Hadland M., 2004. Using Counselling in Mental Health Practice. Chapter 14 In Kirby, S.D., Hart, D.A., Cross, D., Mitchell, G., (eds*). Mental Health Nursing, competences for practice*. Hampshire: Palgrave 178-194.

Hayes, J., Cox, C., 1999. The experience of therapeutic touch from a nursing perspective. *British Journal of Nursing,* 8 (18), 1249-1254.

Henderson, C., Jones, K., 1997. *Essential Midwifery*. London: Mosby.

Hildingsson, I., Häggström, T., 1999. Midwives' lived experiences of being supportive to prospective mothers/parents during pregnancy. *Midwifery,* 15, 82-91.

Hipwell, A. E., Murray, L., Ducournau, P., Stein, A. 2005. The effects of maternal depression and parental conflict on children's peer play. *Child: Care, Health & Developmen,t* 31 (1), 11-23.

Hochschild, A. R., 1979. Emotion Work, Feeling Rules and Social Structure. *The American Journal of Sociology*, 85 (3), 551-575.

—. 1983/2003. *The Managed Heart. Commercialisation of Human Feelings.* London: University of California Press.

—. 2003. *The Commercialisation of Intimate Life, notes from home and work.* London: University of California Press.

Hodnett, E.D., 1999. Support from Caregivers during Childbirth. *The Cochrane Library.*

Hogg, M.A., Vaughan, G.M. 1998. *Social Psychology*, second edition. London: Prentice Hall

Hunter, B., 2001. Emotion work in midwifery: a review of current knowledge. *Journal of Advanced Nursing,* 34 (4), 436-444.

—. 2004. Conflicting ideologies as a source of emotion work in midwifery. *Midwifery,* 20, 261-272.

—. 2005. Emotion work and boundary maintenance in hospital-based midwifery. *Midwifery,* 21, 253-266.

—. 2006. The importance of reciprocity in relationships between community-based midwives and mothers. *Midwifery.* Available from: www.sciencedirect.com (accessed 11/8/06).

Hunter, B., Deery, R., 2009. *Emotions in Midwifery and Reproduction.* Hampshire: Palgrave MacMillan.

Hunter, B., 2009. 'Mixed messages': Midwives experiences of managing emotions. Chapter 10. In Hunter, B., Deery, R.,. *Emotions in Midwifery and Reproduction.* Hampshire: Palgrave MacMillan 175-192.

Husserl, E., 1970. The Crisis of European Sciences and Transcendental Phenomenology. An Introduction to Phenomenological Philosophy. Translated by Carr D. *In*: Moran, D., Mooney, T., eds. 2002. *The Phenomenology Reader.* London: Routledge, 151-174 (Originally published in 1970).

Infant feeding Survey 2000. Available from: www.doh.gov.uk (accessed 6/3/09).

International Confederation of Midwives, 2006. *Essential Competencies for Basic Midwifery Practice.* Available from: www.internationalmidwives.org (accessed 22/5/09).

John, V., Parsons, E., 2006. Shadow work in midwifery: Unseen and unrecognised emotional labour. *British Journal of Midwifery,* 14 (5), 266-271.

Johnson, R., Taylor, W., 2006. *Skills for Midwifery Practice*, 2nd ed. London: Elsevier Churchill Livingstone.

Jones, C., 2002. 1.1 Poverty and Social Exclusion. In Davies, M. (ed). *The Blackwell Companion to Social Work.* Oxford: Blackwell Publishing. 7-19.

Kendrick, K.D., Robinson, S. 2002. 'Tender loving care' as a relational ethic in nursing practice. *Nursing Ethics*, 9 (3), 291-300.

Kirkham, M., 1993. Communication in Midwifery. *In*: Alexander, J., Levy, V., Roch, S., *Midwifery Practice, A research – based approach.* Hampshire: The MacMillan Press Ltd.

—. 1999. The culture of midwifery in the National Health Service in England. *Journal of Advanced Nursing,* 30 (3), 732-739.

—. 2000. *The midwife-mother relationship.* Hampshire: Palgrave MacMillan.

Kirkham, M., Stapleton, H., Thomas, G., Curtis, P., 2002a. Checking not listening: how midwives cope. *British Journal of Midwifery* 10 (7), 447-450.

Kirkham, M., Stapleton, H., Curtis, P., Thomas, G., 2002b. The inverse care law in antenatal midwifery care. *British Journal of Midwifery,* 10 (8), 509-513.

Kirkham, M., 2009. Emotional Work around Reproduction: supportive or constraining? Chapter 13. In Hunter, B., Deery, R.,. *Emotions in Midwifery and Reproduction.* Hampshire: Palgrave MacMillan 227-241

Kitzinger S. 1977. Authoritative touch in childbirth. *In*: Davis-Flyd, R.E., Sargent, C.F., eds. *Childbirth and Authoritative Knowledge: Cross cultural perspectives.* London: University of California.

—. 2006. *Birth Crisis.* Abingdon: Rouledge.

Kitzman, H., Olds, D.L., Sidora, K., 2000. Nurse home visits during pregnancy and early childhood had positive effects on aspects of maternal life course 3 years later. *Evidence based Nursing,* 3, 115.

Klaus M. H., Kennell, J.H., Klaus, P.H., 2002. *The Doula Handbook.* Second Edition. Cambridge: Perseus Publishing.

Kuosmanen, L., Vuorilehto, M., Kumpuniemi, S., Melartin, T., 2010. Post-natal depression screening and treatment in maternity and child health clinics. *Journal of Psychiatric and Mental Health Nursing*. 17, 554-557

Laver, J. 1975. Communicative functions of phatic communication. In Kendon, A., Harris, R.M., Key, M.R., (eds). *The organization of behaviour in face-to-face interactions.* The Hague: Mauton. 215-238

Lawler, D., Sinclair, M., 2003. Grieving for my former self: a phenomenological hermeneutical study of women's lived experience of postnatal depression. *Evidence based Midwifery*, 1(2), 36-41.

Lawrie, T. A., Herxheimer, A., Dalton, K., 2002. Oestrogens and progestogens for preventing and treating postnatal depression. Issue 4. *The Cochrane Collaboration*: Wiley Publishers. www.thecochranelibrary.com

Lazarus, R.S., Folkman, S. 1984. *Stress, appraisal and coping*. New York: Springer

Leap, N., Hunter, B., 1993. *The midwife's tale, an oral history from handywoman to professional midwife*. London: Scarlet Press.

Leininger, M.M., 1985. Transcultral care diversity and universality: a theory of nursing. *Nursing & Health Care*, 6, 209-212.

Lemaitre-Sillere, V., 1998. The infant with a depressed mother: destruction and creation. *Journal of Analytic Psychology*, 43, 509-521.

Lemola, S., Stadlmayr, W., Grob, A., 2007. Maternal adjustment five months after birth: the impact of the subjective experience of childbirth and emotional support from the partner. *Journal of Reproductive and infant psychology*, 25 (3), 190-202.

Leonhardt-Lupa, M., 1995. *A Mother is Born, preparing for motherhood during pregnancy*. London: Bergin & Garvey.

Levy, V., 1999a. Midwives informed choice and power: part 1. *British Journal of Midwifery*, 7 (9), 583-586.

—. 1999b. Midwives informed choice and power: part 2. *British Journal of Midwifery*, 7 (10), 613-616.

—. 1999c. Midwives informed choice and power: part 3. *British Journal of Midwifery* 7, (11), 694-699.

—. 1999d. Protective Steering: a grounded theory study of the processes involved when midwives facilitate informed choices during pregnancy. *Journal of Advanced Nursing*, 29 (1), 104-112.

—. 1999e. Maintaining equilibrium: a grounded theory of the processes involved when women make informed choices during pregnancy. *Midwifery*, 15, 109-119.

Littlewood, J., McHugh, N., 1997. *Maternal distress and postnatal depression*. Hampshire: Palgrave Macmillan.

Logsdon, M.C., Wisner K., Hanusa, B.H., Phillips, A., 2003. Role functioning and symptoms remission in women with postpartum depression after antidepressant treatment. *Archives of Psychiatric Nursing*. 17 276-283.

Lomax, H., Robinson, K., 1996. Asymmetrics in interaction: An analysis of midwife-client talk during the post natal period. Presented at *The International Confederation of Midwives 24th Triennial Congress*, 26-31 May proceedings 252-255.

Lundgren, I., 2004. Releasing and relieving encounters: experiences of pregnancy and childbirth. *Scandinavian Journal of Caring Science,* 18, 368-375.

Lundgren, I., Dahlberg, K., 2005. Midwives' experience of the encounter with women and their pain during childbirth. *In*: Wickham, S., *Midwifery, Best Practice* Vol. 3. London: Elsevier Butterworth Heinmann, 131-140.

Mac Arthur, C., Winter, H.R., Bick, D.E., Knowles, H., Lilford, R., Henderson, C., Lancashire, R.J., Braunholtz, D.A., Gee, H., 2002. Effects of redesigned community postnatal care on women's health four months after birth a cluster randomised controlled trial. *The Lancet,* 359 (Feb 2), 378-385.

Magill-Cuerden, J., 2006. Nurturing and supporting mothers: A hidden skill in midwifery. *British Journal of Midwifery*, 14 (6), 374.

Mann, S., 2004. 'People-work'; emotion management, stress and coping. *British Journal of Guidance and Counselling,* 32 (2), 205-221.

—. 2005. Emotional Labour and stress within mental health nursing. *Journal of Psychiatric and Mental Health Nursing*, 12 (2),154-162.

Mander, R., 2001. *Supportive Care and Midwifery.* Oxford: Blackwell Science.

Mander, R., Reid, L., 2002. Midwifery power. *In*: Mander, R., Fleming, V., *Failure to progress, the contraction of the midwifery profession.* London: Routledge, 1-20.

Marchant, S., 2004. Transition to motherhood: from the woman's perspective. *In*: Stewart, M., *Pregnancy, Birth and Maternity Care, feminist perspectives.* Philadelphia; Elsevier Science, Books for midwives, 71-85.

Marsh, J., Sargent, E., 1991. Factors Affecting the Duration of Postnatal Visits. *Midwifery,* 7, 177-182.

Marxists Internet Archive, 2010. *Encyclopaedia of Marxism.* Available from: www.marxists.org/glossary/frame.htm

McCance, T.V., McKenna, H.P., Boore, J.R.P., 1999. Caring: theoretical perspectives of relevance to nursing. *Journal of Advanced Nursing*, 30 (6), 1388-1395.

McCourt, C., Hirst, J., Page, L.A., 2000. Dimensions and attributes of caring: women's perceptions. *In*: Page, L.A., ed. *The New Midwifery, science, and sensitivity in practice.* London: Churchill Livingstone, 269-291.

McCourt, C., Percival, P., 2000. Social Support in childbirth. *In*: Page, L.A., ed. *The New Midwifery, science and sensitivity in practice.* London: Churchill Livingstone, 245-269.

McCourt, C., 2005. Supporting choice and control? Communication and interaction between midwives and women at the antenatal booking visit. *Social Science and Medicine*, 62, 1307-1318.

McCourt, C., Stevens, T., Sandall, J., Brodie, P., 2006. Working with women: developing continuity of care in practice. *In*: Page, L.A., McCandlish R., eds. *The New Midwifery: Science and Sensitivity in Practice*, 2nd edition London: Churchill Livingstone Elsevier, 141-167.

McCourt, C., Stevens, T., 2009. Relationship and Reciprocity in Caseload Midwifery. *In*: Hunter, B., Deery, R., eds. *Emotions in Midwifery and Reproduction*. Hampshire: Palgrave MacMillan, 17-36.

McCourt, C., 2003. Social support and childbirth, chapter 12 In Squire, C., (ed) *The Social Context of Birth*. Oxford: Radcliffe Medical Press. 187-209.

McGuinness, F., 2006. Defining normal birth would help midwives and mothers. *British Journal of Midwifery*, 14 (6), 328.

McMahon, C., Barnett, B., Kowalenko, N., Tennant, C., Don, N., 2001. Postnatal depression, anxiety and unsettled infant behaviour. *Australian and New Zealand Journal of Psychiatry,* 35, 581-588.

Mercer, R.T., 2004. Becoming a mother versus maternal role attainment. *Journal of Nursing Scholarship,* 36, 226-232.

Miller, A.R., Barr, R.G., Eaton, W.O., 1993. Crying and motor behaviour of six week old infants and post partum maternal mood. *Paediatrics,* 92 (4), 551-558.

Miller, T., 2007. "Is this what motherhood is all about?", weaving experiences and discourse through transition to first-time motherhood. *Gender & Society*, 21 (3), 337-358.

Morrison, V., Bennett, P., 2006. *An Introduction to Health Psychology.* Harlow: Pearson Prentice Hall.

Morrison, P., 1992. *Professional Caring in Practice, a psychological analysis*. Aldershot: Avebury, Ashgate publishing limited.

Morrissey, M. V., 2007. Suffer no more in silence: Challenging the myths of women's mental health in childbearing. *The International Journal of Psychiatric Nursing Research,* 12 (2), 1429-1438.

Morse, J. M., 2001. Towards a Praxis Theory of Suffering. *Advances in Nursing Science,* 24 (1), 47-59.

—. 2000. Responding to the cues of suffering. *Health care for Women International*, 21, 1-9.

Morse, J.M., Bottorff, J.L., Hutchinson, S., 1995. The Paradox of Comfort. *Nursing Research*, 44 (1), 14-19.

Morse, J. M., Bottorff, J.L., Hutchinson, S., 1994. The Phenomenology of comfort. *Journal of Advanced Nursing,* 20, 189-195.

Morse, J. M., Bottorff, J., Anderson, G., O'Brien, B., Solberg, S., 1992. Beyond empathy: expanding expressions of caring. *Journal of Advanced Nursing,* 17, 809-821.

Muniz, A. 2008. *Social Institution of Motherhood; A Brief Historical Overview of Mothering Practices and Ideologies.* Available from: www.suite101.com/content/social-institution-of-motherhood

Murray, L. 1992. The impact of postnatal depression on infant development. *Journal of Child Psychology and Psychiatry*, 33 (3) 543-561.

Murray, L., Cooper, P.J. 1997. Effects of postnatal depression on infant development. *Archives of Disease in Children*, 77, 99-101.

National Childbirth Trust 2010. www.nct.org.uk

National Health Service 2010. NHS careers. Available from: www.nhscareers.nhs.uk

—. 1962. A hospital plan for England and Wales. Cmnd 1604. London: HMSO.

National Institute for Health and Clinical Excellence NHS. 2003. Antenatal care, Routine care for the healthy pregnant woman. *NICE clinical guideline 6.* Available from: www.nice.org.uk

—. 2006. Routine postnatal care of women and their babies. *NICE clinical guideline 37.* Available from: www.nice.org.uk

—. 2007. Antenatal and Postnatal mental health.. Available from: www.nice.org.uk

—. 2008. Antenatal care: routine care for healthy pregnant women. Available from: www.nice.org.uk

Nelson-Jones, R., 1995. *The Theory and Practice of Counselling*, 2nd ed. London: Cassell.

Newell, S.J., Miller, P., Morgan, I., Salariya, E., 1997. Management of the new born baby: midwifery and paediatric perspectives. *In*: Henderson and Jones eds. *Essential Midwifery.* London: Rooutledge, 229-265.

Ngai, F-W., Chan S.W-C., Ip, W-Y., 2009. The effects of a childbirth psychoeducation program on learned resourcefulness, maternal role competence and perinatal depression: A quasi-experiment. *International Journal of Nursing Studies.* 46, 1298-1306

Norman, I., Ryrie, I., 2009. *The Art and Science of Mental Health Nursing, a text book of principles and practice*, second edition. Berkshire: McGraw Hill, Open University Press

Nursing Midwifery Council, 2004. *Codes of Conduct for Nurses and Midwives.* London: NMC.

—. 2008. *Codes of Conduct for Nurses and Midwives*. London: NMC.
—. 2009. *What does a midwife do?* Available from: www.nmc-uk.org (accessed 5/6/09).
Oakley, A., 1988. Is Social Support good for the health of mothers and babies? *Journal of Reproductive and Infant Psychology*, 6 (1), 3-12.
—. 1992. *Social Support and Motherhood.* Oxford: Blackwell Science.
Oakley, A., Rajan, L., Grant, A., 1990. Social Support and Pregnancy Outcome. *British Journal of Obstetrics and Gynaecology,* 97, 155-162.
Oats, J. 1994. *The Foundation of Child Development.* Oxford: Blackwell / Open University.
O'Cathlain, A., Walters, S.J., Nicholl, J.P., Thomas, K.J., Kirkham, M., 2002. Use of evidence based leaflets to promote informed choice in maternity care: randomised controlled trial in everyday practice. *BMJ,* 324, 643-6.
Ogden, J., 2000. *Health Psychology, a textbook.* Second Edition. Buckinghamshire: Open University Press.
Ólafsdóttir, Ó. Á., 2009. Inner knowing and Emotions in the Midwife-Woman Relationship. *In*: Hunter, B., Deery, R., eds. *Emotions in Midwifery and Reproduction.* Hampshire: Palgrave Macmillan, 192-210.
Olds, D.L., Robinson, J., O'Brien, R., Luckey, D.W., Pettitt, L.M., Henderson, C.R., Rosanna, K.N., Sheff, K.L., Korfmacher, J., Hiatt, S., Talmi, S., 2002. Home visiting by paraprofessionals and by nurses: a randomised controlled trial. *Paediatrics* 110 (3), 486-496.
Olds, D.L., Kitzman, H., Cole, R., Robinson, J., Sidora, K., Luckey, D.W., Hanks, C., Bondy, J., Holmberg, J., 2004. Effects of nurse home visiting on material life course and child development: Age 6 follow-up results of a randomised trial. *Paediatrics,* 114 (6), 1550-1559.
Page, L.A., 2000. Keeping birth normal. *In:* Page, L.A., ed. *The New midwifery, science and sensitivity in practice.* London: Churchill Livingstone, 105-123.
Page, L.A., McCandlish, R., 2006. *The New Midwifery, Science and Sensitivity in Practice*, 2nd ed. Philadelphia: Elsevier.
Pairman, S., 2000. Women-centred Midwifery: Partnerships or Professional Friendships? *In*: Kirkham, M., ed. *The Midwife-mother relationship*. London: MacMillan Press Ltd., 207-225.
Papalia, D.E., Olds, S.W., Feldman, R.D., 1998. *Human Development*, seventh edition. New York: McGraw Hill.

Pemberton, C., 2010. Will Social Workers lose their touch? *Community Care*. August. www.communitycare.co.uk

Phipps, B., 2005. Normal birth – does it matter? *In*: Wickham, S., *Midwifery best practice* vol. 3. London: Elsevier Butterworth Heinemann, 140-143.

Rhodes, P., 1995. *A short history of Clinical Midwifery*. Cheshire: Books for midwives press.

Richards, J., 1999. *Caring for People, a lifespan approach*. Cheltenham: Stanley Thornes (publishers) Ltd.

Roberts, R., Towell, T., Golding, J.F., 2001. *Foundations of Health Psychology*. Hampshire: Palgrave.

Robertson, A., 2000. Pregnancy and birth – sexy? You bet! *The Practicing Midwife*, 3 (8), 34-5.

Robinson, K., Lomax, H., 1996. Exploring the midwife-client relationship: A new analytical perspective. Presented at the *International Confederation of Midwives 24th Triennial Congress*, 26-31 May proceeding pages 252-255.

Rogers, C. R., 1951. *Client Centred Therapy*. London: Constable.

Rothman, B.K., 2000. *Recreating Motherhood*. New York: W.W. Norton & Company

Royal College of General Practitioner, 2010. General Practice. www.rcgp.org.uk

Rowan, C., McCourt, C., Bick, D. 2010. Provision of perinatal mental health services in two English strategic health authorities: views and perspectives of the multi-professional team. *Evidence Based Midwifery*. Vol. 8 No 3, 98-106

Rungapadiachy, Dev. M., 1999. *Interpersonal Communication and Psychology, for health care professionals, theory and practice*. Oxford: Butterworth Heinemann.

Sagrestano, L.M., Feldman, P., Rini, C.K., Woo, G., Dunkei-Schetter, C., 1999. Ethnicity and Social Support During Pregnancy. *American Journal of Community Psychology*. Vol. 27, No 6, 869-898

Sandell, J., 1997. Midwives' burnout and continuity of care. *British Journal of Midwifery*, 5 (2), available from: www.intermid.co.uk (accessed 11.05.07).

Savage, J., 2004. Researching emotion: the need for coherence between focus, theory and methodology. *Nursing Inquiry*, 11(1), 25-34.

Schuiling, K.D., Sampselle, C.M., 1999. Comfort in labor and midwifery art. Image: *Journal of Nursing Scholarship*, 31 (1), 77-81.

Schott, J. 2005. Parent Education: meeting the needs of fathers. In Wickham, S. (ed.). *Midwifery, Best Practice Volume 3*. London: Elsevier Butterworth Heinemann

Shields, N., Reid, M., Cheyne, H., Holmes., McGinley, M., Turnball, D., Smith, L.N., 1997. Impact of midwifery-managed care in postnatal period: an exploration of psychosocial outcomes. *Journal of Reproductive and Infant Psychology*, 15 (2), 91-108.

Sidebotham, M., 2004. NICE guideline: antenatal care under the microscope. *British Journal of Midwifery*, 12 (3), 137-140.

Sinclair, D., Murray, L., 1998. Effects of Postnatal Depression on Children's Adjustment to School. *British Journal of Psychiatry,* 172, 58-63.

Skinner, G., 2005 Action: promoting normal birth. *In:* Wickham, S., ed. *Midwifery best practice* vol. 3. London: Elsevier Butterworth Heinemann, 143-145.

Smith, M. 2004. Review of research related to Watson's Theory of Caring. *Nursing Science Quarterly*, 17 (1), 13-25.

Smith, P., 1992. *The Emotional Labour of Nursing, how nurses care*. Hampshire: MacMillian Press Ltd.

Stapleton, H., Kirkham, M., Thomas, G., 2002a. Qualitative study of evidence based leaflets in maternity care. *BMJ,* vol. 324 March.

Stapleton, H., Kirkham, M., Thomas, G., Curtis, P., 2002b. Midwives in the middle: balance and vulnerability. *British Journal of Midwifery,* 10 (10), 607-611.

Stapleton, H., Kirkham, M., Curtis, P., Thomas, G., 2002c. Framing information in antenatal care. *British Journal of Midwifery,* 10 (4), 197-201.

Stewart, M., 2004. Pregnancy, Birth and Maternity Care, feminist Perspectives. London: Elsevier, Books for Midwives.

Stickley, T., Freshwater, D., 2002. The art of loving and the therapeutic relationship. *Nursing Inquiry*, 9 (4), 250-256.

Strongman, K. T., 1996. *The Psychology of Emotions*, fourth edition, theories of emotion in perspective. Chichester: John Wiley & Sons.

Suttie-Gunson, R., 2007. What makes a Good Mother? *Parenting* Nov 12th. Available from: www.parenting.youk.com (accessed 27/2/09).

Sykes, J. B., (ed) 1982. *The Concise Oxford Dictionary of current English, seventh edition*. Oxford: Clarendon Press.

Tammentie, T., Tarkka, M., Kurki, A., Paavilainen, E., Laippala, P., 2004a. *Journal of Psychiatric and Mental Health Nursing,* 11, 141-149.

Tammentie, T., Paavilainnen, E., Astedt-Kurki, P., Tarkka, M., 2004b. Family dynamics of postnatally depressed mothers – discrepancy between expectations and reality. *Journal of Clinical Nursing,* 13, 65-74.

Taylor, M. C., 2005. Interviewing. *In*: Holloway I. ed. *Qualitative Research in Health Care.* Berkshire: Open University Press, 39-53.

Teti, D.M., Gelfand, D.M., Messinger, D.S., Isabella, R. 1995. Maternal depression and the quality of early attachment: an examination of infants, preschoolers, and their mothers. *Developmental Psychology,* 31, 364-376.

Tew, M., 1998. *Safer childbirth? A critical history of maternity care.* London: Free Associate Books

Thurgood, M., 2009. Engaging clients in their care and treatment. Chapter 27. In Norman, I., Ryrie, I., (eds). *The Art and Science of Mental Health Nursing, a text book of principles and practice*, second edition. Berkshire: McGraw Hill, Open University Press, 621-637.

Walsh, D., 1999. An Ethnographic study of women's experience of partnership caseload midwifery practice: the professional friend. *Midwifery,* 15, 165-176.

Waterhouse, L. 2002. 1.3 Child Abuse. In Davies (ed), *The Blackwell Companion to Social Work,* 2nd edition. Oxford: Blackwell Publishing.

Way, S., 2000. *Core skills for Caring and Assessment.* Midwifery Practice Guide 7. Manchester: Books for midwives.

Whitton, A., Warner, R., Appleby, L., 1996. The pathway to care in postnatal depression: women's attitudes to post natal depression and its treatment. *British Journal of General Practice*, 46 (408), 427-428.

Wickham, S., 2005. *Midwifery, Best Practice* vol. 3. London: Elsevier Butterworth Heinemann.

Wilkins, C., 2006. A Qualitative study exploring the support needs of first-time mothers on their journey towards intuitive parenting. *Midwifery,* 22, 169-180.

Wilkins, R., 2000. Poor relations: The paucity of the Professional Paradigm. *In*: Kirkham M ed. *The Midwife-mother relationship.* London: MacMillan Press Ltd., 28-52.

Williams, C., 2004. Midwives and sexuality: earth mother or coy maiden. *In*: Frith, L., Draper, H., eds. *Ethics and midwifery*, 2nd ed. London: Elservier Science, 110-127.

Williams, A.M., Irurita, V. F., 2004. Therapeutic and non- therapeutic interpersonal interactions: the patient's perspective. *Journal of Clinical Nursing,* 13, 806-815.

Wolf, N., 2001. *Misconceptions.* London: Chatto and Windus.